BUSINESS/SCIENCE/TECHNOLOGY DIVISION
CHICAGO PUBLIC LIBRARY
400 SOUTH STATE STREET
CHICAGO, IL 60605

D0847454

Chicago Public Library

REFERENCE

Form 178 rev. 1-94

SportsMedicine

for the

Combat Arts

By

Joseph J. Estwanik, M.D.

Publisher's Cataloging in Publication

Estwanik, Joseph J.
  SportsMedicine for the combat arts / Joseph J. Estwanik, M.D.
  p. cm.
  Includes index.
  LCCN: 96-83747
  ISBN: 1-888926-00-7

  1. Martial Arts 2. Boxing 3. Aerobics 4. Fitness
  5. Grappling 6. Wrestling 7. Law Enforcement Training
  8. Sports Medicine I. Title

RC1210.E78 1996   617.1'027
                               QBI96-20236

All rights reserved.

Copyright 1996 ©

No part of this book may be reproduced or transmitted in any form
or by any means, electronic or mechanical, including photocopy-
ing, recording or by any information storage and retrieval system
without permission from the publisher.

Published in the United States of America

Boxergenics™ Press

Delmar Printing Company

Charlotte, North Carolina

R01212 11104

BUSINESS/SCIENCE/TECHNOLOGY DIVISION
CHICAGO PUBLIC LIBRARY
400 SOUTH STATE STREET
CHICAGO, IL 60605

NOTICE TO READERS

Boxergenics™ Press is now accepting original book manuscripts. If you are interested in submitting an original manuscript for review and possible publication, please forward to:

Boxergenics™ Press
335 Billingsley Road
Charlotte, NC 28211

Or you may call (704) 334-4663 or
toll-free 1-800-774-6284 for further information.

Dedication

I wish to thank all of those dedicated physicians, coaches, and officials who selflessly serve as advisors, "father-figures," and friends to the many youth seeking guidance; not only in the combat arts and confines of the ring, but along the open pathway of life. Their countless hours of dedication humbly pale my ringside and book writing experiences. Thanks to my uncomplaining family.

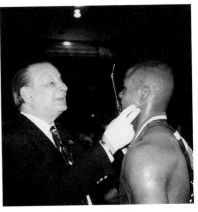

Dr. Necip Ari with boxer

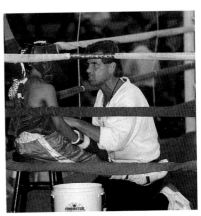

Coach Tom Moraetes with boxer

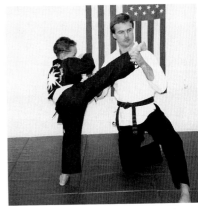

Master Irwin Carmichael with martial arts student

SportsMedicine for the Combat Arts

(Martial Arts, Boxing, Grappling, Wrestling, Law Enforcement)

Chapter 3

Chapter 11

Chapter 12

Chapter 13

Chapter 14

Chapter 15

Chapter 16

Chapter 17

Chapter 18

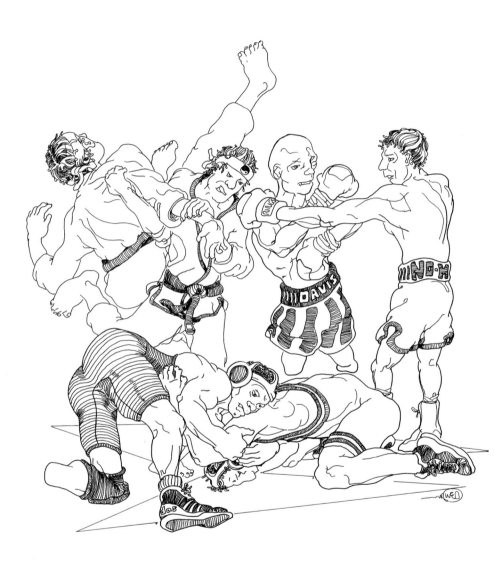

About the Author

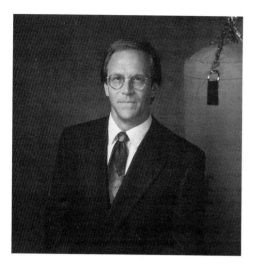

Sportsmedicine physician and orthopaedic surgeon Dr. Joe Estwanik hasn't missed a week of weight training for 36 years. When he's not practicing medicine, he might be bicycling, jogging, hiking, camping, pistol shooting, practicing martial arts, doing boxing aerobics or even open-water kayaking in a typical week. He has also acted as a ringside physician for the past 15 years, actually supervising over ten thousand boxing bouts.

The North Carolina-based doctor was tending to the sports injuries of a professional soccer team when he was asked to be a ringside physician at the USA Boxing National Championship event in Charlotte, North Carolina, in 1981. He was surprised to learn that boxing as a sport was "stuck in the Dark Ages." "It seemed to be completely divorced from the academic milieu of sportsmedicine," Estwanik recalls. "I've been heavily involved since then in making positive contributions to the sport by incorporating the current principles and practices of modern sportsmedicine."

He has elevated the academics of the combat arts to such a level that he now is chairman and organizer of an annual **Ringside Physician's Course** located within the U.S. Olympic Training Center, Colorado Springs. His annual courses became international in scope with both instructors and participants arriving from foreign countries. All profits generated by the course are donated to USA Boxing. Dr. Estwanik has organized his experiences and recommendations into three separate chapters within a 1995 medical textbook, *Boxing and Medicine,* edited by Robert Cantu, M.D.

His expertise in disseminating down-to-earth and practical sportsmedicine wisdom to the general public has made him a frequently solicited speaker. Dr. Estwanik's 79 broadcasts on WBT radio's ***Injuries of the Week*** and 31 appearances on WSOC TV's ***Midday Healthbeat*** have honed his relaxed yet enthusiastically sincere demeanor. Quotes by the "doc" in *USA Today, Detroit Free Press, Dallas Daily News, Black Belt, Fitness, Shape,* and *US Air* magazines have substantiated his dominance as "the source" for safety and fitness.

Formerly the National Medical Chairman for USA Boxing's Junior Olympic Boxing Program, Dr. Estwanik was appointed Chairman of the Sportsmedicine Committee for USA Boxing, allowing close, productive communication with coaches, athletes, and officials.

As the founder of **Boxergenics™,** the first "boxing-for-fitness" exercise video program to be endorsed by United States Amateur Boxing, Inc., the national governing body for Olympic-style boxing, 49-year-old Dr. Estwanik is the creator of an exercise regime that effectively blends the techniques of

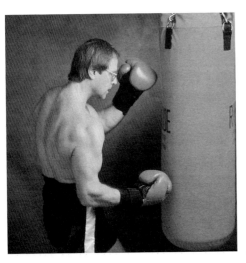

boxing, the discipline and respect of martial arts, the fitness benefits of aerobics, and the injury prevention of sportsmedicine. Dr. Estwanik will soon release a textbook, *Boxergenics™,* highlighting five chapters on basic boxing technique based on interviews with five former Olympic level coaches.

Sensing a definitive need to better protect the hands of his favorite athletes, Dr. Estwanik holds two patents on high tech gloves which are now being marketed and distributed. "It is a shame that competitors wrap their hands by the same methods used over 200 years ago. My designs apply the use of modern biomaterials and biomechanical principles to protect the hand of the puncher as well as we now protect the foot of the runner." **The Corepad™ Handwrap®** will protect the hand and wrist during training while the **Grappling Glove®** will benefit the competitor.

Experience as a safety consultant and ringside physician has positioned him into his consulting ringside physician duties for ***Battlecade Extreme Fighting, World Combat Championships,*** and ***Ultimate Fighting Championships.***

Dr. Joe Estwanik studied orthopaedic surgery at The Cleveland Clinic and Bowman Gray School of Medicine of Wake Forest University in Winston-Salem, North Carolina. His dedication to amateur boxing has taken him all over the world, including Moscow, London, Paris, and Bombay. He currently resides in Charlotte, North Carolina with his wife, Janice, and their three children and balances his athletic pursuits by teaching nature photography.

Acknowledgements

I wish to thank the following for their assistance and contributions
to this book:

Publicist and Vice-President of Marketing: Brenda Loyed Coley

Proof-Readers: Nancy Yudell Segal, R.N., B.S.N., M.A.T. and
William A. Primos, M.D.

Illustrator: William E. Davis, R.N.

Carolina Health Physical Therapy: Greg Cates, P.T., Franz Foster,
P.T., Tim Cates, P.T.A., Beth Ahlers, A.T.C., Lynn Hughes,
A.T.C., Robin Simmons

Delmar Printing and Publishing Company: Ed Bohannon and Sherrie Atwell

Cover Photograph: Winston-Salem / Forsyth County Schools

Ballet Photograph: Courtesy of Danella Bedford, Charlotte School
of Ballet

USA Judo Photographs: Scott Gardener, A.T.C., Nashville, TN

U.S.A. Boxing, Inc.

My Instructors: Master Irwin Carmichael, Grand Master Bobby
Taboada, Grand Master Remy Presas, George Mandrapilias

My Teachers: Dr. George Rovere—Bowman Gray School of
Medicine, Dr. H. Royer Collins—The Cleveland Clinic Foundation, Dr. John Bergfeld—The Cleveland Clinic Foundation.

Mouth Guards: Courtesy of John Gaetano, President, Tuf-Wear

Focus Pads: Courtesy of John Brown, President, Ringside Products

Heavy Bag: Courtesy of John Brown, President, Ringside Products

Contributors

Richard Birrer, MD
Chairman, Dept. of Emergency
Medicine
Catholic Medical Center of Brooklyn &
Queens, Jamaica, New York
and
Associate Professor, Dept. of Medicine
Cornell University, New York, NY
and
Panel Physician
New York State Athletic Commission
and
Editor, *SportsMedicine For The Primary
Care Physician,* Second Edition

Robert C. Cantu, MA, MD
Chief, Neurosurgery Service
Director, Service of Sports Medicine
Emerson Hospital, Concord, MA
and
Medical Director
Nat'l Center for Catastrophic Sports
Injury Research
and
Editor, *Boxing And Medicine*

Frank P. Filiberto, MD
Chief, Otolaryngology Division
Dept. of Surgery
Sebastian River Medical Center,
Sebastian, FL

William A. Primos, MD
Chief, Primary Care SportsMedicine
Metrolina Orthopaedic SportsMedicine
Charlotte, NC

Lacey Walke, MD, MS, FRCS(C)
Asst. Professor of Anatomy and Cell
Biology
Wayne State University School of
Medicine, Detroit, MI
and
Senior Surgeon
Bon Secours Hospital, Grosse Pointe,
MI
and
Chief, Section of General Surgery
Macomb Hospital Center, Warren, MI

Donald Ralph Werner, MD
Adjunct Professor of Ophthalmology
New England College of Medicine
Biddeford, ME
and
Ophthalmologist
Brighten Medical Center, Portland, ME
and
Medical Director
Maine State Athletic Commission
and
Team Physician
USA National Water Polo Team

Disclaimer

This text was designed to provide information on the subject matter covered. It is sold with the understanding that this author and the publisher are not rendering exact medical, injury, or organizational advice. Medicine and the treatment of sports injuries are not exact sciences, but a highly subjective art. If medical assistance is required, without delay, seek the services of a competent professional.

The purpose of this text is to assemble pertinent facts and situations useful to devoted athletes, coaches, instructors, and parents. Please read other related source books, involve your coaches, and do not neglect or minimize any injury. It is your responsibility to seek professional advice in a timely manner.

Because of individual human variation, circumstances of injury, level of competition, age, and pre-existing factors, a second and third opinion may be advisable.

Every effort has been extended to provide accurate and experienced opinion. However, there **may be mistakes** both typographical and in content. Treatment recommendations and medical advances create an environment of change. This text is only a general guide for a diverse group of athletes and not the ultimate recipe for complicated problems.

The purpose of this text includes education and entertainment. The author and Boxergenics™ Press shall have neither liability nor responsibility to any person or entity with respect to any loss or damage, or alleged to be caused, directly or indirectly by the information contained in this text. If you do not wish to be bound by the above, you may return this text to the publisher for a full refund.

Introduction

My personal commitment to the medical care of athletes involved in the combat arts has rewarded me with many friends. Irwin is a multi-talented law enforcement officer (also a martial arts instructor) who represents the Mecklenburg County Sheriff's Department in womens safety awareness classes and has authored a book entitled *Women's Awareness Response*. The didactic portion of each session evolves into practical tactics that highlight his crafty demonstration of self-defense moves. In one intended slow-motion demo, a hyped and tense student rapidly and unexpectedly kneed this master instructor in the head as he bent over to show the class a common attack position. He was k.o.'d but quickly, and most embarrassingly, expedited the graduation of all in attendance so as to end the class. He appeared in my office the next day still a little woozy, nauseated, and headachy. Neurologic exam was safely negative for serious neurologic involvement. My concluding diagnosis was post-concussion headache requiring rest and limited physical exertion. Only one problem—he was entered in a full contact martial arts tournament in five days and the entrance fee was already paid. Because our bonds of trust were built on solid information, experience, and sincere interest, my advice was readily and unquestionably accepted. He sat this one out! Womens self-defense, law enforcement training, and martial arts competition all encompass the combat arts.

Rick has been a favorite patient for many years. I have counseled Rick through his many wrestling injuries as he competed in free-style tournaments even after the completion of a college career. Knee, shoulder, and elbow injuries kept him a frequent patient. Rick had finally aged into the role of coaching my own children in the art of wrestling at their junior high school. Coach Rick was prematurely struck down by a stroke that had no known relationship to a sports activity. In fact, his unbelievable athletic ability, fitness level, and tenacity enabled him to resume coaching activities despite losing his eyesight for objects occupying his left field of vision. A temporary loss of driving privileges didn't rob him of his independence as he resolutely either jogged or bicycled to teach school each day. Rick still rolls on the mat and coaches state champion athletes. These dedicated athletes of the mat deserve the best of information that Combat Arts Sportsmedicine can supply. USA Wrestling, our Olympic Federation for wrestling, estimates that approximately 120,000 youths annually pursue training in this scholastic grappling art. The recent sky-rocketing interest in the martial-arts-driven World Com-

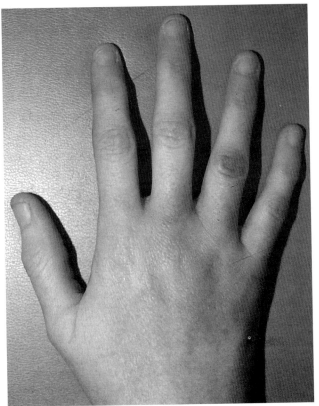

bat Championships, Extreme Fighting, and Ultimate Fighting Championships undeniably catapults into reality the effectiveness of grappling as a major combat tool. Many institutions of traditional martial (not marital) arts forms are seeking the expertise of wrestlers (grapplers) to supplement their training experiences.

Linda was a first time patient with a big time swollen hand. In her interest to gain fitness, she purchased the

Figure I-A: Notice bruising from inadequate padding and technique

equipment, but not the knowledge. In the pursuit of an aerobic boxing workout, she hung the new heavy bag in her doorway, donned the most flimsy excuse for a glove, failed to protectively wrap her hands, and knew no punching techniques. Her very first powerfully misguided punch (Figure I-A) ricocheted off the side of the bag and into the wooden door jam. Her "handy work" was a result of improper equipment, technique, and instruction! Luckily, x-rays demonstrated that no fractures and no tendons were permanently injured. I think her hand healed far faster than her ego. The growing legions of aerobic boxers who employ these techniques for fitness, muscular symmetry, self confidence, weight loss, and self defense are patients worthy of sportsmedicine advice specific to the Combat Arts.

Calvin is a dedicated college student busily studying within the College of Business Administration. He doesn't drink. He doesn't party all night. He eats, sleeps, and trains as a boxer, in fact, an elite boxer with the ranking of #4 in the United States. Studious and intelligent as he is, injuries still creep up within his well-planned training program. His powerful punch has created exces-

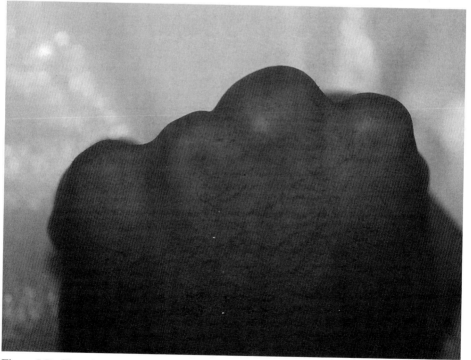

Figure I-B: Chronic MCP joint inflammation typical in punchers. New protective handwraps are now available.

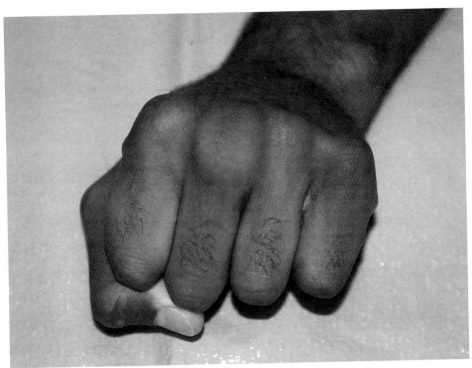

Figure I-C: Boxer's knuckle indicating chronic MCP joint inflammation.

sive pressure upon his long finger MCP (knuckle) joint. (Figures I-B and I-C) Pain and swelling threaten to limit his workouts and endanger his competitive ranking. A special problem in a special athlete! Unfortunately, this is an all too common affliction.

Appropriate handwrap techniques, therapy, injections, and medications are allowing him to pursue his lofty and realistic aspirations towards the Olympic Trials. Indeed, special treatment skills become necessary in serving this dedicated youth, a role-model within the Combat Arts. USA Boxing confirms that 21,659 are competing within their well established and structured programs. The explosion of fitness boxing, aerobic boxing, and Boxergenics™ by the "white collar" and fitness crowd creates a vast uninformed group.

Pete, a law enforcement trainee, must become somewhat proficient in restraint techniques. His familiarity in these tactics and skills is glaringly scrutinized by the press. Brutal techniques are out and more humane control methods are demanded. These demands, however, place the officer himself at a greater risk of personal injury both in training and real-life application. Our "community's best" deserve a new and understandable source of informative sports injury reference. Likewise, many fire fighters employ martial arts exercises to remain fit during their 24 hour "on call" shifts in our nation's complex of fire stations. An authoritative sportsmedicine text will keep them on the streets and up the ladders.

It is estimated that 8 million U.S. citizens are actively pursuing martial arts training. Women, seeking fitness and concerned with their personal safety, comprise 25% of USA participants. They are the most rapidly growing segment. (Figure I-D) Youth commonly train in the arts, also capturing another 25% of the total. Men frequently seek competitive tournaments, often with full contact rules. I have volunteered as medical care for youth tournaments that only allow less intense "point fighting." Minor injuries have occurred nevertheless, and awareness of injury treatment concepts will benefit all ages of participants.

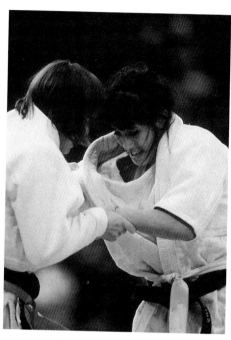

Figure I-D: Women in martial arts — the fastest growing segment

These Forgotten Many comprise an astoundingly large population of athletes whose pursuits are nonspecifically ignored by traditional, classic sportsmedicine concepts. A deficiency of safety and injury treatment advice leaves participants clamoring for experienced and factual expertise.

My pertinent experiences include:
1. Orthopaedic surgeon specializing in sportsmedicine.
2. National Chairman of the SportsMedicine Committee, USA Boxing.
3. Appointment by my governor to The North Carolina State Boxing Commission.
4. Ringside physician experience in over 10,000 bouts including exotic locations in Moscow, London, Paris, Bombay, and critical events includ-

ing world championships, Olympic trials, and the Goodwill Games.

5. Consulting ringside physician for the Ultimate Fighting Championships, Extreme Fighting, and World Combat Championships.

6. Lecturer in sportsmedicine for the U.S. Wrestling Federation in the early 80's.

7. The author of three significant, scholarly, published research articles about wrestling injuries within the medical literature.

8. A physician for the U.S. Olympic Wrestling trials in the 70's.

9. A high school wrestler in the 60's.

To assist all worthy participants I feel a "voluntary" obligation to share information with these tremendously dedicated athletes. My personal and professional interactions confirm their deep appreciation for guidance, expertise, and experience. My respected professor, Remy A. Presas (Modern Arnis) taught me that in the most noble of martial arts and coaching tradition, we must *"SHARE THE KNOWLEDGE."*

For any dubious historical importance, a portion of this text was written during my "quiet time" as a volunteer physician at the United States Olympic Training Centers (Lake Placid, New York and Colorado Springs, Colorado) and in my room at the sport hotel that housed athletes for the 1994 Goodwill Games in St. Petersburg, Russia. St. Petersburg lies so far north in Russia that my daylight lasted until nearly midnight during our mid-July competitions. My duties as team and ringside physician for boxing provided a unique perspective into the inner motivations, personal adaptations, team dynamics, work ethics, and leisure time of our elite USA (and foreign) boxers. I'll always consider it an honor to have been included and accepted as a "team" member. Outstanding coaches! Talented athletic representatives from my country! When viewing the great discipline and dedication they expended in the performance of their art, I am humbly challenged to equally apply my healing arts.

The star high school football quarterback must literally restrict the doctors standing in line to treat him while the boxer, wrestler, or martial artist frequently finds himself silently sitting at the edge of the mat, in the locker room or a corner of the training dogo shaking his/her head wondering what to do next.

All of these athletes share a disciplined hunger for knowledge in injury prevention, treatment, and rehabilitation. I am compelled not to starve these motivated men, women, and youth.

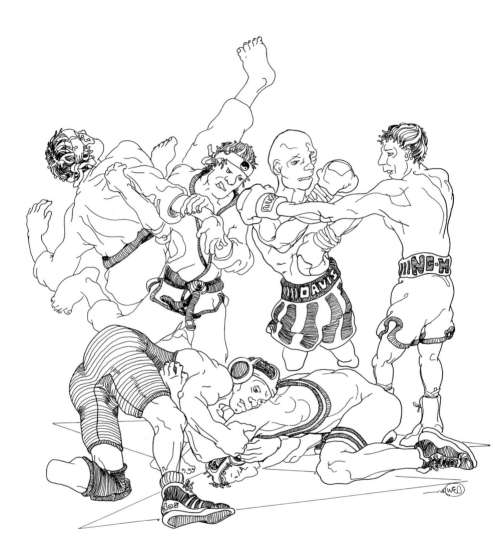

Chapter 1

The 10 Rules
for Ringside Observation
(Monitoring Safety)

M any years of observing the ups and downs of competitors from ringside has allowed me to establish 10 practical monitoring hints. All of my comments may not be based on researched, academic calculations; just experienced, real-life, solid basics.

"I CAN'T SEE HIS EYES, BUT I CAN WATCH HIS *FEET.*"

1. STANCE—a confident stance directly relates to that participant's skill level and training efforts. Balance means everything! A flat-footed, wide based posture infers either an inadequately prepared novice or an injured fighter. The progression to a staggering stance denotes head injury or other major problems.

2. RING MOVEMENT—Here's our chance to view "poetry in motion." The art and grace of athletics is no more evident than the floating, skillful movements of a dominant athlete. Without consulting scoreboards, computers, or bout sheets the winner can be reliably predicted by who "dominates" the action. The "running" boxer is the defeated boxer (unless far ahead in points and purposefully avoiding the taking of risks). You can just about base your score on the gross positioning of competitors.

"I CAN'T SEE HER EYES, BUT I CAN WATCH HER *HANDS.*"

3. DEFENSE—The big "D." This third principle actually occupies the #1 safety priority and reigns supreme for safe and timely cessation of com-

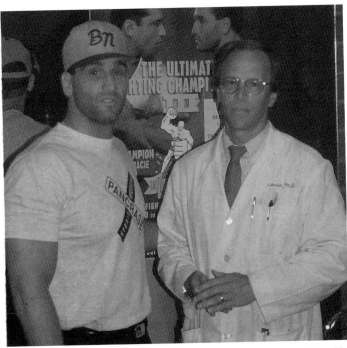

Figure 1-A: Dr. Estwanik serving as head physician for The Ultimate Fighting Championships pictured with Ken Shamrock, Winner of UFC #3

petition. An effective defense is the ***ultimate determinate*** for combat safety. When defense is absent the bout, match, or contest must cease. A winner has already emerged. In 1979, Dr. I. A. McCown wisely stated, "A one-sided contest should be halted minutes early, rather than seconds late." This mirrors my mind-set and is readily quoted when potentially opening myself to criticism for demanding that a bout be stopped.

4. PUNCH COUNT—The active and busy competitor is rarely in trouble. When a boxer is throwing punches, a wrestler working for the pin, or a martial artist creating combinations, we know that they remain healthy. Again, a winner can be predicted merely by—'Who is throwing?' and 'Who is busy?'.

5. LOWERED ARMS—Unless one possesses a very unconventional style, the sign of lowered arms means trouble. Fatigue and accumulated body blows will take their toll and drop the arms—thus opening the athlete to dangerous head blows. Boxing coaches urge patience and instruct the fol-

lowing pattern of attack to their athletes—"GO TO THE BODY AND THE HEAD WILL FOLLOW." Knowledgeable audiences also understand the concept of "working the body" as I have amusingly heard them shout—"TAKE THE TIRES OFF THAT TRUCK." Sometimes, elbows are lowered to protect injured ribs. At times an injured extremity necessitates a one-armed contest. More than once, I have intently followed, for a round or two, a boxer who slyly shields an injured shoulder, elbow, or hand as he protects his lead to hang-on for the win. If his defense remains adequate, I'll hang on to the edge of my seat with him.

FATIGUE FACTORS

6. CLINCHES—It is no surprise that tired athletes "tie-up" an opponent to slow the flow of action. A tired, winning wrestler will ride his opponent while failing to work for additional points or a pin. Out of interest, I have counted the number of tie-ups or clinches within boxing events. In Reality Fighting, these 5 or 10 situations per round would have provided excellent opportunities for a grappler to bring the boxer to the ground and

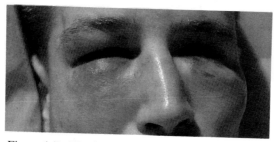

Figure 1-B: "Bruise news" — accumulating trauma

into foreign territory for warfare. (Figure 1-A)

7. "BRUISE NEWS"—ACCUMU-LATING TRAUMA—If an athlete is just plain getting "beat up" and accumulating facial swelling, small cuts, bruises, bloody nose, etc., the writing is on the wall. Usually, the winners stay pretty, but extremely competitive bouts may equally dole out the punishment. (Figure 1-B)

8. NUMBER OF STANDING "8" COUNTS—The "standing 8 count" is a tremendous addition to the safety controls within the combat arts. All competitions should seek to add this referee

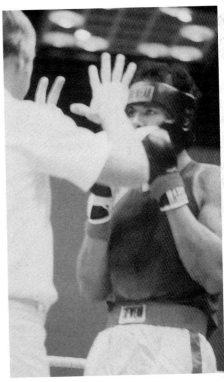

Figure 1-C: Standing "8" Count

option. Amateur boxing rules stipulate defeat when a boxer receives three "8's" in a single round or a total of four "8's" during the bout. It is a good rule. Getting the "8" saves athletes from the impending knockout and ceases one-sided contests. (Figure 1-C)

EXTRANEOUS FACTORS

9. REFEREE LEVEL OF ATTENTIVENESS—If a *competent* referee is handling the bout, the worries of the doctor, coach, parent, and athlete can be eased. If a skilled referee is hyper-alert to one athlete, hovering close to break up the action, moving in tight to peer into his eyes, watch out! If good referees are nervous, I am nervous. If bad referees aren't nervous, I am nervous. Their level of activity and attentiveness mirrors the flow of action and concern. (Figure 1-D)

10. CORNER ACTIVITY—Nobody should know the athlete better than his personal coach. Focusing on the coach's facial grimaces, smiles, intense

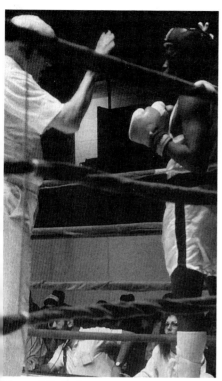

Figure 1-D: Referee's level of attentiveness

posture, or relaxed body imaging, tells the tale of the tape. If they're happy, I'm usually happy. If they focus hyperactive attention to a cut or extremity during the one minute rest periods between rounds, I have an insider's hint on which stock to buy—what area to observe during the next round. If you get to know the coaches, you'll better learn to accurately read their body language. (Figure 1-E)

By understanding and utilizing my 10 Rules for Ringside Observation, as a parent, coach, referee, or doctor, (Figure 1-F) you'll accurately predict winners, losers, and injuries. By alertly following a bout, I estimate a 90%+ accuracy level in predicting the injuries that will be present as competitors exit

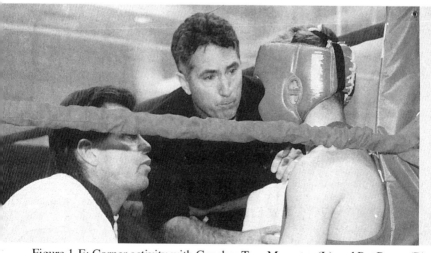

Figure 1-E: Corner activity with Coaches Tom Moraetes (L) and Pat Burns (R)

from the ring. However, sports and the art of medicine will be forever humbling. Just when you think that you know it all, the ever-motivated loser lands a lucky punch and knocks out his overwhelmingly superior opponent or the wrestler quickly reverses and pins his opponent.

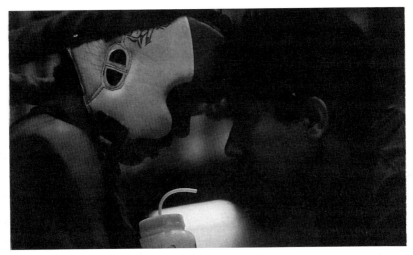

Figure 1-F: Father and son

Chapter 2

The Essential Basics

FLEXIBILITY

You know the hype, I've seen the ads. *"Kick high, kick cold, kick butt!"* I don't easily forget the martial arts magazine advertisement for a stretching rack—*"Don't be limited!"* The trademark, the goal, the status, the image of an effective martial artist has been hyped with high kicks. Frequent ads, biased interviews, and multitudes of misinformation fill the pages of karate magazines. Must you kick high to be good? What are the limits of stretching? Can we change ourselves past the usual benefits obtained with a good warm-up and thorough flexibility program? Has anyone bothered to quote references or scientifically monitor research to document the hype? I ran a computerized medical literature search called **MEDLINE** to gather such studies relative to hip movement in karate. Guess what? They don't exist. I suspect more money has been spent on the correct consistency of peanut butter than the medical effects, frustration levels, and secondary injuries of countless wasted hours of groin stretch. Magazine ads support the need to achieve this end point with no regard to scientific documentation or research dollars spent. The martial arts magazines reader is over-powered by high flying endorsements to split wide and kick high. Much energy has been wasted, many frustrations (not kicks) are heightened, and more potential for injury is proliferated by these teasers. Some people, many people, were not internally designed to pattern their training as advertised.

For many years, I examined martial arts students who sought treatment at our Sportsmedicine Clinic for training or competition injury. Having tested and documented numerous hip ranges of motion for martial artists, I have arrived at the conclusion that advanced belt levels do not necessarily correlate with increased ranges of hip motion. If stretching lacks some natural endpoint and promises unlimited individual barriers, shouldn't all experienced, devoted masters of the art have achieved extremely supple and similar end results? Power, speed, accuracy, and technique are the proper standards by which to train and seek improvement. Unwarranted movement past the obtainable goals of warm-up and flexibility of the soft tissues can be hazardous. Compare the goal of "kick high" in the martial artist to the achievement of turn-out or the "first position" in the ballerina. A scientific research study of hip problems in ballet quite shockingly suggests some very contemplative statistics. In their 1989 study, *"Degenerative Joint Diseases in Ballet Dancers"* Swedish physicians Andersson and Nilsson found the incidence of hip arthritis among dancers "significantly higher than the general population." Others do argue that the conclusion of "arthritis being produced by extreme physical activity" is unfounded and not supported by any data. But, should we subject our hips to forces that are extraordinary? Ballerinas, at an early age, obtain "turn out" by actually altering and stretching their hip structures. Have you ever watched an elite ballerina walk? You will notice that

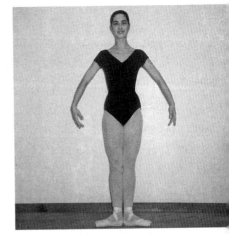

she has sacrificed the ability to walk normally, standing and walking with her feet rotated constantly outward, like a duck. This is a significant and permanent price to pay for performance and "the look." (Figure 2-A)

Utilizing 21 intermediate to advanced level male martial artists, I:

1. Measured their ability to perform a "Chinese" split (legs out to the sides, instead of the "American" split with one leg forward and one leg to the rear).

Figure 2-A: Ballerina in "turn out" — Danella Bedford, trained at The Royal Ballet School, United Kingdom

2. Documented their actual range of hip motion.

3. X-rayed their hips and pelvis while in the split.

4. X-rayed their pelvis and hips in a routine neutral position.

5. Requested a questionnaire on their stretching habits, goals, and personal impressions of being flexible or tight.

From measuring their x-rays in every conceivable manner, I attempted to understand if there was a primary structural factor allowing "high kickedness." Disappointedly, no single major breakthrough was uncovered, but several clarifications did emerge.

1. My manual measurements of hip movement and x-ray techniques were accurate and consistent.

2. We discovered a trend to suggest that the shape of one's hip is a relevant factor in hip flexibility. We are pursuing a greater number of participants IN THIS STUDY to increase the statistical significance.

3. The athlete's ability to rotate his hip outward (external rotation) does allow one to "cheat" into a wider split or higher kick.

Remember that every martial arts participant was not created and designed equally if we limit our discussion to kicking high. Human anatomical variation dictates the extremes of movement sorted out to individuals. Our goals should be realistic and individualized. Should a shot-putter risk his scholarship on additional aspirations of putting in those miles to become a marathoner? Likewise, can a slightly-built long distance runner ever expect to perform admirably as a shot-putter, much less vigorously train for this event without expecting injury? Our athletes should not unrealistically pursue non-anatomic "turn out" or split by extraordinary measures, not to exclude good common-sense stretch programs, in order to attain higher rank. We suspect that forced movement has created disability in older ballerinas. There might be a costly price to pay! Thankfully, the myriad of martial arts styles allows extreme variety in choosing training patterns, tempo, intensity, and arm-leg movements. This is a great thing! Not everyone has to become a high kicker, nor should they doggedly train to become so. Just "let it happen!"

And back to those ads—***"Kick high, kick cold, kick butt!"*** Not all of us were made to kick high—accept that fact! When one performs without a proper warm-up, as in an emergency, we do have an increased chance for injury and there is no way around that. Choose your own personalized style. You don't have to kick high to kick butt. In fact, I would consider kicking to the butt as low and safe, but a questionably effective target.

"Don't be limited" also has its limits. We are all limited. We all have our strong points and weak points. Utilize and perfect those strong points while cautiously working around and compensating for your inherent weaknesses.

WARM-UP

Don't confuse warming-up with stretching!

What is **the** perfect workout and training session? The answer to that inquiry has no more universal conclusion than an argument about your favorite automobile or star athlete. There are, however, basic components to a scientific, well planned program that are firmly established and not "fair game" to criticize. Relying heavily on my background in orthopaedic surgery, I'll dissect the skeleton of an accepted workout session. Don't confuse warming-up with stretching!

A full body **warm-up**, "break a sweat" or "break a bead," **before** stretching initiates the proper sequence as warming up a muscle promotes greater stretching gains and less chance for injury. A **warm-up** actually increases your body's core temperature. This rise is only achieved from activities like jumping jacks, jogging, and bicycling. A stretch program does not actually warm you up for the increased challenges of a sporting activity. In fact, stretching is most effective only after you are "warmed up." So let's get the sequence in proper order:

1. Warm-up

2. Light stretch program

3. Workout or weight training

4. Major stretch program
   * (Include 2 - 3 strength training workouts per week.)

STRETCHING

Stretching is one of the most **misunderstood** concepts among athletes, instructors, and the general public. Most participants don't stretch correctly and end up wasting their time, missing effective end results and often injure themselves unknowingly. Timing is everything. Despite tradition, recent research recommends that the majority of your stretch effort occur towards the end of a workout. By placing major stretching emphasis at the conclusion of a vigorous training program, accumulated lactic acid can be flushed from the muscles resulting in less "sore muscle syndrome" the following day. Your exercised muscles will recover faster if all the breakdown products can escape.

A proper stretch program can fulfill the goals of:

1. Improved range of motion

2. Enhanced performance

3. Less muscle soreness after workout

4. Prevention of injury

"Pain" triggers a warning system for our brain. It pulls the fire and burglar alarms to sound in our head. Painful stretch can be one of these intruders. Your body does not want you to hurt yourself and supplies many natural responses to noxious stimuli. Pulling aggressively on muscle only fires up the fibers within that muscle and actually contracts, rather than relaxes, the structures that you are targeting to stretch. "No pain—no gain" is archaic and has no application to stretching programs. Perform your stretch movement until a firm tightness with slight discomfort is felt. If you relax and hold steady at that position—lengthening of that muscle complex will occur. Progressively increase that same stretch.

The ineffective, bad, injurious type of old-fashioned bounce stretch is called **ballistic stretch.** Avoid it! It doesn't work because the more rapidly an elongating force is applied to a muscle complex, the greater is that tissue's resistance to stretch. I'll "pull out" my taffy pulling analogy. If you slowly pull on taffy, it will stretch and stretch and stretch. Pull on taffy quickly and it breaks abruptly. Be sweet to your muscles while stretching. "Go to all lengths" to provide non-ballistic methods of stretch.

An article "Guidelines for Proper Stretching" by Ninos in the February 1995 *Journal of Strength and Conditioning* details two types of correct stretch as (1) static stretch and (2) proprioceptive neuromuscular facilitation stretch.

1. **Static stretch** is that effective slow stretch that has been preached with some regularity. The newest of research suggests that a single stretch with a 30-second minimum is necessary for an actual lengthening of musculotendinous units. In other words, you must, in a relaxed position, place the muscle in its maximally lengthened position and hold it there for a 30-second minimum with three to five repetitions being necessary. (Figure 2-B)

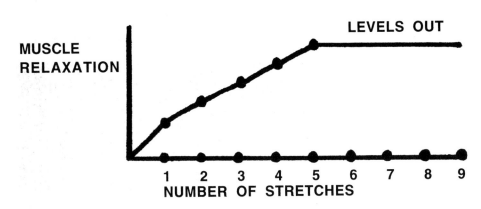

Figure 2-B: Stretch effectiveness graph

Let's get practical! The hamstring is a useful muscle to explain these facts of life. The competitor should stretch the left hamstring for 30-seconds and then focus his efforts into a 30-second stretch on the right side. Go back to the left and then the right. Now do this a third and and final time. We have devoted a 3-minute minimum time period to the important hamstring area. I know that you are thinking—"I don't have hours to devote to stretch," or "I need to use my valuable and limited time for …". My practical suggestion is to:

(a) understand your sports demands,

(b) know your own body, and,

(c) factor-in previously injured areas of your anatomy.

With these three areas recognized, you then focus upon the major muscle groups that most require your attention. Stretch every day but vary the routine. Work the units of major stress daily and add in less important units on a rotational schedule.

2. **P.N.F. stretch** (proprioceptive neuromuscular facilitation) is better understood as contract/relax or hold/relax than stretch. Once you get past this intimidating name and learn about this extremely useful system of alternating contraction and relaxation of the targeted muscle and its antagonist muscle, you will accelerate gains. This technique is performed with a knowledgeable partner and can be amazingly effective. (Figure 2-C) Its sequence for stretching the hamstring is explained in Figure 2-C.

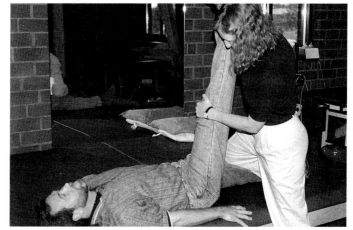

Figure 2-C: P.N.F. (proprioceptive neuromuscular facilitation) stretch for hamstrings.

CONCLUSIONS AND ILLUSTRATION OF TECHNIQUES

1. **Do** stress the fundamentals of warm-up for all body parts—upper body, trunk, and lower limbs.

2. **Do** perform stretches that relax and lengthen the specific soft tissues challenged by a workout. For example, don't forget the shoulders before and **after** punching.

3. **Do** allow solo and cautious partner stretching patterns.

4. **Do** understand the difference between BALLISTIC (bad, **bouncing, harsh**) and STATIC (smooth, controlled, slow motion) stretches. The individual movements of stretch need to be held **30 seconds** to be effective. The majority of effective muscle tissue lengthening occurs after the first 3 to 5 stretches. Great time and effort spent in excess of 3 - 5 **slow** stretches is inefficient and nonproductive.

5. **Do** allow some free time for personalized stretches so that participants can focus upon individual areas of tightness or prior injury. Not all students need to spend equal time on similar body parts. Some are naturally "looser" than others and many have prior injury patterns that they need to focus upon.

6. **Do** allow a major stretch session as a post exercise "cool down."

7. **Do** seek reliable instruction in the advanced stretching technique called P.N.F.—"Proprioceptive Neuromuscular Facilitation." Once you get past this intimidating name and learn about the extremely useful system of alternating contraction and relaxation of the targeted muscle and its antagonist muscle, you will accelerate gains.

8. **Do not** force a joint into unnatural positions of excess flexion or excess extension. (Figure 2-D)

9. **Do not** apply great leverage to obtain results. (Figure 2-E)

10. **Do not** allow the effects of gravity to be utilized as a leverage force, i.e., perform most stretches on the mat rather than standing or leaning over. (Figure 2-F)

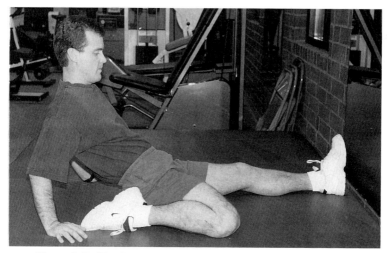

Figure 2-D: Hurdler's stretch. Excessive pressure on the knees

11. **Do not** generally perform rotational exercises on susceptible body parts such as the neck, low back, and knees. (Figure 2-G)

12. **Do not** use another's body weight to force a stretch.

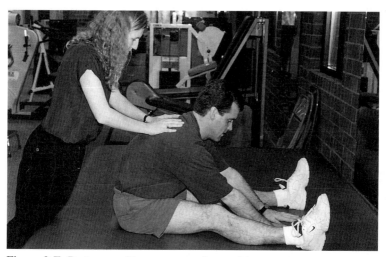

Figure 2-E: Partner pushing someone forward in seated split. Excessive pressure not controlled by the athlete. Too much leverage.

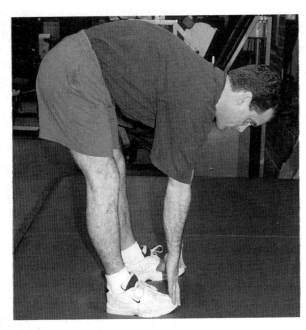

Figure 2-F: Standing toe touch. Excessive pressure on the spine. Negate gravity's forces by sitting.

13. **Do not** forget to include upper extremity stretches in your warm-up routine. (Figures 2-H, 2-I, 2-J, 2-K)

14. **Do not** stretch to the point of pain. If a stretch causes pain, an involuntary reflex causes your hurt muscle to contract in an effort to pull away from the painful stimulus—you!

15. **Do not** stretch unstable joints, such as a previously dislocated shoulder, unless supervised by a sports physician or physical therapist.

16. **Do not** enter into an aggressive stretch program on a previously injured body part—such as a bad low back—until your program is designed by a doctor or therapist.

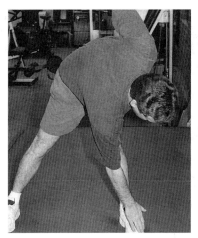

Figure 2-G: Trunk rotation — Excessive forces exerted when standing

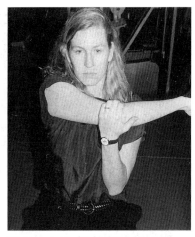

Figure 2-H: Shoulder stretch — Good positioning

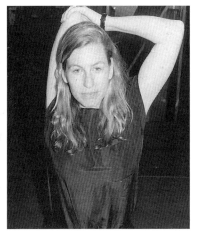

Figure 2-I: Shoulder stretch — Proper positioning

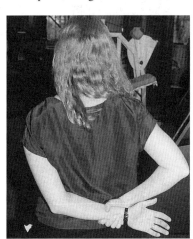

Figure 2-J: Shoulder stretch — Proper form

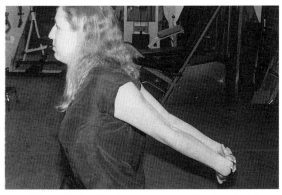

Figure 2-K: Shoulder stretch — Useful stretch

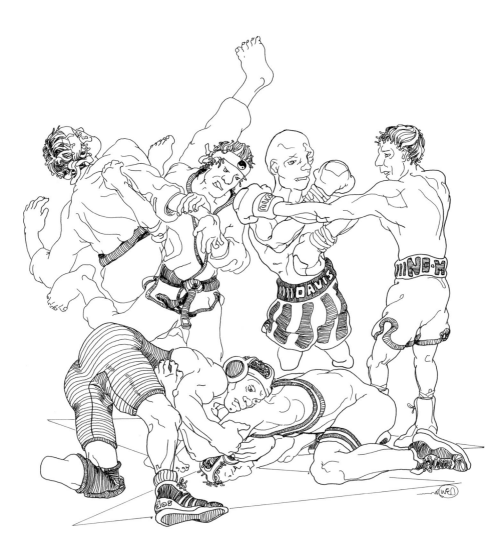

Chapter 3

Hand & Wrist Injury

INTRODUCTION

The joints, bones, ligaments, and tendons of the hand can become injured in any number of ways. Dr. Charles Melone, noted hand surgeon for the pros in New York City, has described the known forces of a punch as follows:

1. Axial Compression—a direct blow

2. Angular Forces—missed or misdirected punches

3. Excess Tension—we microscopically sublux our knuckle joints at impact

Although wrestlers and martial artists expose their open hands, fingers, feet, and toes to numerous mechanisms of potential injury, boxers (with a closed fist) limit their common sites of trauma. Boxers consolidate injury to:

1. Traumatize MCP joints of index and long fingers

2. Impact the carpal-metacarpal joints of index and long fingers to cause arthritis (metacarpal-carpal bossing) (Figure 3-A-1 and Figure 3-A-2)

3. Catch the thumb in an awkward position as the collateral ligament is sprained (gamekeeper's thumb)

4. Suffer a variety of metacarpal fractures

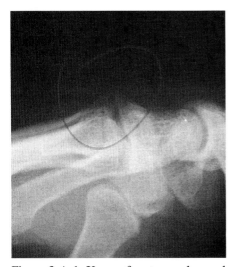

Figure 3-A-1: X-ray of metacarpal-carpal bossing

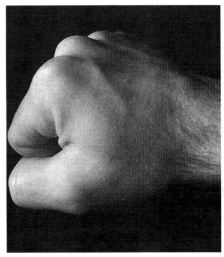

Figure 3-A-2: Photo of metacarpal-carpal bossing

DIP (DISTAL INTERPHALANGEAL) FINGER JOINT

The DIP (distal interphalangeal) joint is the finger joint closest to your fingernail. It definitely works only as a hinge joint (in 1 plane) and allows no side-to-side or rotational movements. Proper range of motion encompasses fully straight (0°) to full flexion of 90° (a right angle). (Figure 3-B)

MECHANISM

A quite common injury to this most distal joint occurs with an excessive bend into flexion which tears the extensor tendon. The common names for this injury include "baseball" finger and "mallet" finger. Maybe martial artists can name this "spear-hand" finger. The names are rather graphically explanatory! As the ball player attempts to catch a ball, it arrives too soon and hits the top of the finger before he can fully open his hand to catch the ball with the palm surface.

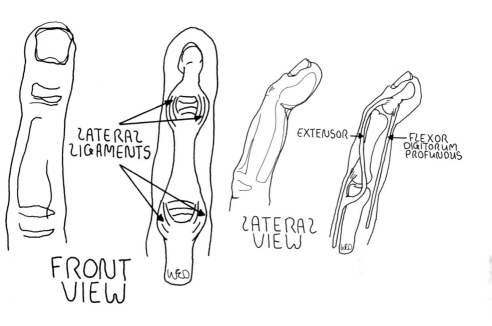

Figure 3-B: Lateral ligaments and flexor digitorum profundus

DIAGNOSIS

Mallet finger describes the resulting deformity as the extensor tendon tears and the tip of the finger droops into flexion. The athlete is ***no longer able*** to straighten this joint because the connections have been torn. (Figure 3-C)

Sometimes the force of the bend will even pull off a piece of bone where the tendon anchors. UNLESS this piece of bone constitutes a significant portion of the joint surface, this accompanying small fracture can be ignored and treated just like the tendon injury. The mechanism of the bone injury is identical—a sharp bending force that either tears the tendon lose or uproots the tendon with a portion of its anchoring bone. X-rays are important so that your doctor can confirm whether a fracture has occurred and, most critically, whether the bone forms a sizable portion of articulating joint surface.

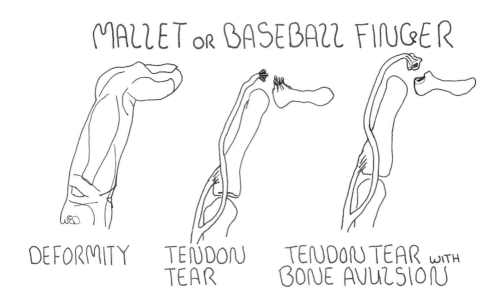

Figure 3-C: Drawings of deformity, tendon tear, bone fragment

TREATMENT

"The sooner the better!" If you position that finger into full extension by means of a splint, and hold it there **CONSTANTLY** for 6 weeks, it will usually heal. However, let's emphasize several points.

1. The joint must be held in full extension (fully straight) so that the recently torn ends will meet and have a chance to glue themselves together again.

2. There are several convenient splints on the market.

3. Your doctor must periodically evaluate your skin to be certain that subtle prolonged pressure from the splint does not quietly erode and kill your skin. I have seen this complication occur in patients who failed to keep appointments and wondered WHY their finger was beginning to smell in the splint.

4. **CONSTANTLY** was capitalized because it constitutes a "capital crime" if you remove your splint and let the finger drop at any time during the

six week healing period. Delicate strands of uniting scar are forming between the disrupted ends of the tendon. **IF** you pull these ends apart prematurely before the "glue sets up" and the scar matures, the sequence is ruined. Your healing response has been stalled-out never again to regain its momentum.

5. An x-ray will assist your doctor's decision whether a fracture fragment is large enough to deserve surgery. Usually, splinting alone ALLOWS a small fragment to lie close enough to its origin that perfect re-alignment is unnecessary and meddlesome. Function will be better than the final x-ray.

6. Don't expect a perfect cosmetic result. Do expect a small bump and a slight droop. Your ability to fully use the finger will exceed the slight "war wound."

7. Expect some early stiffness for several weeks to months as you come out of the splint. With time your bend will likely improve. If you "improve" too soon, stretching out of the newly repaired tendon might occur. Be a patient patient!

FLEXOR TENDON INJURY

Although not too common in the combat arts, the flexor tendon can be torn loose from its palm-side moorings. (Figure 3-D) Likewise, occasionally a piece of anchoring bone is also pulled loose.

MECHANISM

In football players this injury is termed "jersey finger." Not with a capital "J," but referring to a player grasping an opponent who pulls away while this finger is caught in a jersey "shirt," a martial arts uniform, or entangled in any piece of equipment. The sudden pulling away on a flexed and contracted tendon rapidly pops loose its attachment.

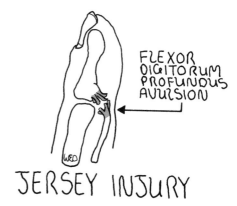

FLEXOR DIGITORUM PROFUNDUS AVULSION

JERSEY INJURY

Figure 3-D: Flexor digitorum profundus avulsion

DIAGNOSIS

An inability to curl the tip of the finger into a full arc provides a warning. X-rays are useful to rule out associated bone injury—realizing that tendons themselves and other soft tissues DO NOT SHOW on plain old x-rays.

TREATMENT

Open surgery is necessary to re-attach this tendon. Because of muscle contractions, this avulsed tendon is pulled so far away from its origin that there is no hope of re-attachment without surgical assistance. Sorry! Significant grip strength will be lost if you don't seek assistance. Six to eight weeks of closely-monitored fancy splints will follow the surgical repair.

PIP FINGER JOINT

A finger dislocation is a very common athletic injury and usually occurs a the PIP (proximal interphalangeal) joint. (Figure 3-E and Figure 3-F) Don' most of us know stories of a competitor or coach who has pulled a finger back into place when a gross deformity occurred? (Thus the name "coach's finger." In these common situations, the ligaments do unfortunately tear, but luckily critical tendons usually remain intact.

Remember:

A. **Ligaments** attach bones to bones.

B. **Tendons** attach contractible muscles to bones. (Figure 3-G)

MECHANISM

An improperly angled force, which loads and torques the joint, tears throug the complex of encompassing ligaments and usually forces the finger into th position depicted.

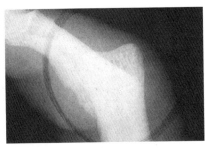

Figure 3-E: PIP (proximal interphalangeal) joint dislocation

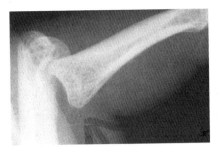

Figure 3-F: PIP (proximal interphalangeal) joint dislocation

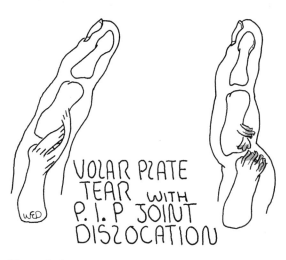

Figure 3-G: Volar Plate tear with PIP joint dislocation.

TREATMENT

If medical care is close, please let your doctor treat this injury. If not, apply longitudinal traction to reduce the overlapping bones allowing them to "pop" back into place. X-rays are useful to confirm the absence of fracture and assure a proper diagnosis! I have found that once a joint is reduced back into normal alignment, small chips that were camouflaged by the deformity might be recognized. Their presence may not change treatment but can foretell the ease or difficulty of healing. The presence of a significant amount of associated bone fracture within the joint changes this injury from "common" into a complicated, permanent problem.

CASE HISTORY

Jim Handler, an attorney, was playing volleyball one Sunday afternoon when a powerful and direct shot was spiked into his unprepared and unpositioned hand. His left little finger suddenly got a little bigger in circumference as the classic dislocation (with no fracture) occurred. I met him in the emergency room and after appropriate x-rays, I applied the highly professional "big pull." After a few grunts and inappropriate legal jargon, the smile returned to his face. Jim is a very competitive and active outdoorsman and had pledged to attend a scheduled golf tournament 10 days away and counting. He agreed to "buddy taping" and a dorsal splint. As the story goes, he did play golf but taped his little finger to both his long and ring fingers as some insurance to benefit his golf grip. Upon interrogation six months following the injury, he recalls having gained full movement about 30 days after the injury. He has since paddled many raging rivers and parred many a hole. A slight loss of full extension is present if one critically analyzes his finger. Understand that if you have broken into the joint surface, and a significant step-off or irregularity is present—proper restoration is necessary. Surgery may be required. "Whatever it takes" is the rule!

Some dislocations will cause excess scarring to deposit around the volar plate. If the volar plate adheres to the bone, a troublesome flexion contracture (loss of ability to passively straighten this joint) may require a surgical release. Each case must be individually analyzed.

MCP (METACARPOPHALANGEAL) FINGER JOINT (Figure 3-H)

We must protect the knuckles. Long term abuse of the fist, the hand, and the knuckles will devastate the day-to-day function of the hand, much less, the opportunity to utilize the hand for healthy fitness activities. The hand is very much taken for granted and not appreciated for the very intricate duties we ask of it. It's simple—yet complex. An injury to a small joint of the hand is just as problematic as an injury to a larger joint. Recovery time is often just as extensive as injuries to the ankle or knee. Just because we are dealing with **little** joints—don't assume we have a little problem. The only compensation is the luxury of owning 10 fingers and the option to utilize some substitution

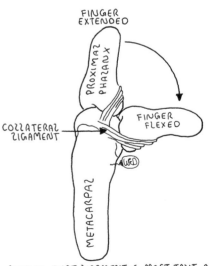

Figure 3-H: MCP (metacarpophalangeal) joint

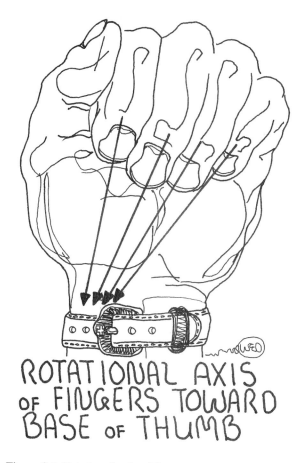

ROTATIONAL AXIS OF FINGERS TOWARD BASE OF THUMB

Figure 3-I: Rotational axis of finger towards base of thumb

techniques that aren't available when having one of two knees or one of two ankles injured. What simple things doesn't the average person appreciate about the hand? The thumb is extremely important to the total overall usefulness of your hand. Should you suffer the loss of your thumb in a disastrous accident—you will have a 50% disability (disabling loss of function) of the entire hand. Each and every finger is designed to "oppose" or push against your thumb. Close your fist, one finger at a time, and you will see that each fingernail is aimed, not straight downward, but within a similar axis aimed towards the base of your thumb. (Figure 3-I)

The index and long fingers comprise the **precision** side of the hand and when joined with the thumb are used for writing, threading a needle, or accurate movements in the work shop. This is due to the fact that these three fingers form the stable,

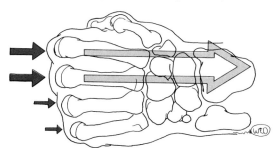

PROPER PUNCHING FORCES onto HAND

Figure 3-J: Proper punching forces onto hand

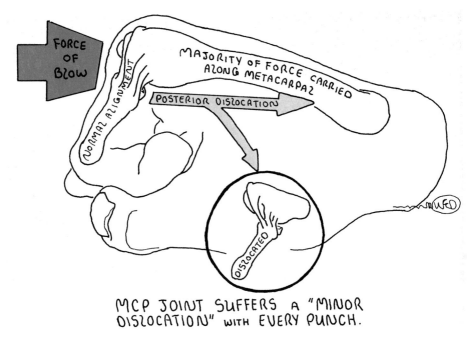

MCP JOINT SUFFERS A "MINOR DISLOCATION" WITH EVERY PUNCH.

Figure 3-K: MCP joints suffering "A Minor Dislocation" with every punch

steady portion of the hand. The index and long finger metacarpals are locked onto our wrist and remain very solid, a reason why we punch with these two knuckle joints. Their stability provides a bedrock for precise movements. (Figure 3-J) The ulnar side of the hand—the ring and little fingers—form the **power** side of the hand. They are mobile and can wrap around objects like a barbell, hammer, or rope. Try grasping a hammer strongly and only use two fingers in the process. I guarantee the most conforming and secure power grip will be formed with the more supple ring and little fingers.

Protect your knuckles. The MCP joints suffer a "minor dislocation" every time you contact or punch a bag. (Figure 3-K) If not supported and cushioned many of these miraculous ligament structures will fatigue and break. A metal hanger used properly and for its purpose will perform its duty as a hanger for a lifetime. If we inappropriately bend it back and forth, back and forth, 40 or 50 times at the same spot, it will fatigue and break. This is the identical mechanism for injury applicable to the boxer's knuckle or the stress fracture in the runner's leg. God and nature can miraculously heal if we give ourselves suf-

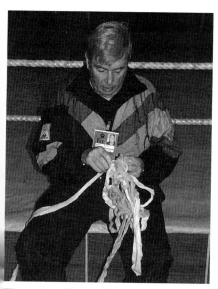

Figure 3-L: Former Olympic Coach Tom Coulter untangling old fashioned hand-wrap materials

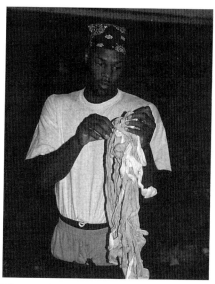

Figure 3-M: Elite boxer Benjamin McDowell wasting time as he untangles handwrap materials

ficient time to heal and repair. If we overpower, abuse, or overuse the system—a noticeable injury appears. Assistive devices such as the COREPAD™ handwraps utilize modern shock absorption materials to lessen impact forces and stabilize at-risk joints. No longer are inconvenient, ineffective, 14 foot layered cotton wraps the only alternative. (Figures 3-L, 3-M, 3-N) If the runner's feet deserve to be protected by the most modern of materials, it is now time to apply those same biomaterial advances to the hand. (Figure 3-O) Utilize the Corepad™.

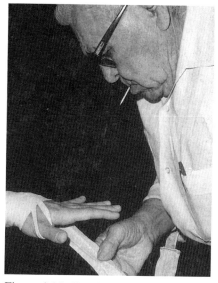

Figure 3-N: Coach Lou Kemp applying handwrap

EXTENSOR TENDON RUPTURES

I served as ringside physician on a getting-down-to-brass-tacks trip to the former Soviet Union in 1988. Our U.S. team was fine-tuning its final shake-

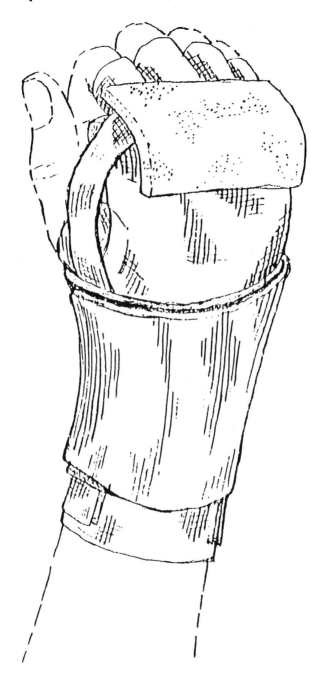

BOXERGENICS COREPAD HANDWRAP™®
1-800-774-6284

Figure 3-O: Corepad™ Handwrap

down stages in preparation for the Seoul Olympics. The energy and excitement that emanated from "performing" before a uniformed Soviet-soldier thick crowd in a huge coliseum warmed our mid-March Moscow trip. Incidentally, this particular event, U.S.A. vs. U.S.S.R. in 1988, was hosted by the then intact Soviet Union. The first of our two competitions was held in a massive Moscow arena over-flowing with enthusiastically patriotic Russsian soldiers. Our 15 member U.S. delegation represented a most insignificant percentage of the cheering crowd! We became a tiny red, white, and blue island within a massive red sea. The largest goose-bump, chest-puffing, heart-throbbing proud seconds of my life were imprinted when our National Anthem reverberated throughout the respectful Cold war crowd. Our arch enemies demonstrated well disciplined class. The realities of boxing were a dull second to this honor!

Riddick Bowe, our then recognized U.S. super heavyweight champion, was toe-to-toe with his always tough Soviet counterpart. Each team was field testing and polishing their expected Olympic team favorites. With each amateur athlete boxing his three rounds (unless decisively stopped early), Riddick unexpectedly stopped throwing combinations in the middle of the second round. His third round was gamely fought one-handed. After his narrow defeat, I removed his handwrap in our Soviet locker room to discover that he was unable to straighten his finger. He had punched the Russian so solidly in the early second round that he literally tore the capsule that anchored an extensor tendon directly over the central axis of a knuckle (MCP joint). This tendon was sitting dislocated into the valley between two knuckles causing a total loss of its pulley-like mechanical advantage. I manipulated this spaghetti-like structure back to its home on the mountain top of the metacarpal head and then tightly taped two gauze sponges into those valleys on either side to prevent redislocation. To complete the story, surgery was eventually performed. Riddick Bowe did win a silver medal losing to Canada's Lennox Lewis in the finals. He entered The Olympic Games not quite 100% healed and not at his fittest.

HAND FRACTURES

Three goals must be satisfied when treating any fracture to a bone in the hand.

1. Each **smooth** articular (joint) surface must be maintained, or arthritis develops.

2. The **length** of each bone must be preserved. Any significant shortening leads to muscle-tendon imbalances resulting in deformity, weakness, lost movement.

3. A broken bone must heal in its original axis of **rotation**. Malrotation is unacceptable. If rotated or spiraled towards the thumb or little finger side of your hand, the twisted finger will always be in the way as you attempt to close your fist.

JOINT SMOOTHNESS

A fracture (break) occurring at either end of a bone is far different than an injury along the shaft. Once a fracture of the **shaft** of a bone has healed in appropriate position—the job is done. Simplistically, the shaft of a bone is simply a stable strut to support its joints, muscles, tendons, and ligaments (the moving parts). Each joint must travel in a full, smooth arc of motion. A stiff or arthritic joint hurts and causes disability. The joints of the hand are intricate and don't tolerate a displaced fracture line. Only an x-ray can properly evaluate the smoothness of joint surfaces. Required restoration of the articular surface follows the dictum—"by any means necessary." If it takes a manual manipulation, cast, pins, or screw—do it. There is most definitely a "golden period" for reduction of deformity within a joint—"the sooner the better." A surgeon encounters great difficulty with repairing a displaced bone segment already stuck down by callous. Fresh edges are much easier to match together. Try completing a puzzle with its edges chewed-up, dissolved, or missing. A fully restored, glass-smooth articular surface has a fighting chance to regain full movement if properly timed, and modern physical therapy is coordinated with recovery.

LENGTH

Even though x-rays highlight only bone, don't forget that many other crucial structures travel alongside this x-ray—visible strut. Just because adjacent soft structures aren't easily imaged, don't overlook them and concentrate only on bone. These vital soft tissues are supported by that calcium-rich strut. Muscle-tendon units and ligaments are designed to operate within certain tensile strengths, lengths, and coordinated linkages. If a bone is significantly shortened by injury, it is no longer maintaining these balances along its full length. The tendons that flex our fingers may be out of sync with those that extend. As a result, a fixed deformity of flexion or extension (bending or straightening) could develop. Not every bone in the hand and finger is equally critical in this respect, so seek expert advice from a jock doc, orthopaedic surgeon, or hand specialist.

ROTATION

Let's get one thing straight—you don't need crooked fingers. The index (pointer) finger can get you into trouble if it doesn't live up to its name. Many fractures occur as a result of a twisting motion which creates a long 3-D spiral pattern of fracture rather than a simple transverse crack. (Figure 3-P) When setting a fracture, one must be certain that each injured finger maintains its proper rotatory alignment.

Recently a patient came to my office in a temporary splint applied in the emergency room. His hand and fingers were held incorrectly (although temporarily) in the fully extended position—as if shaking a hand. His long finger, metacarpal shaft fracture, was obliquely spiraled. Only when bent his MCP (knuckle joints) into about 70° flexion did it appear obvious that the plane of his fingernails didn't properly line-up. The fingernail of his long finger was rotated well

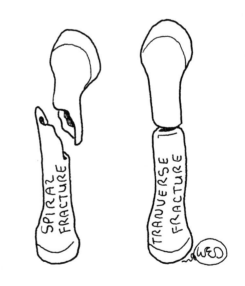

Figure 3-P: 3-D spiral pattern of fracture rather than simple transverse crack

away from the same orientation as the other fingers. In fact, that flexed finger was aiming across his palm rather than in the identical axis of its neighbors. A manipulation of this fracture was needed. Buddy-taping to the adjacent index and ring fingers guarded against further loss of alignment and a cast was applied with the MCP (knuckle) joints flexed to 70°. A significant disability exists when a misaligned finger crisscrosses the others while attempting to grasp an object.

An expert must advise and treat you. A broken finger can be disabling and its unwise "macho" to tape it yourself and suffer the consequences. A powerful grip and agile finger movements are keys to many hand techniques in self-defense.

THUMB

Don't let it all hang out. Keep your thumb folded into and over your fist. (Figure 3-Q) Injuries occur when the "hanging-out-there" thumb is forced away from the hand by an opponent's punch or hooking onto the bag as a punch is thrown. Ligaments are torn if the forces become too great, placing stressed joints at a mechanical disadvantage. Most commonly, this classic injury is called a "gamekeeper's" thumb. In snow country this same injury results from

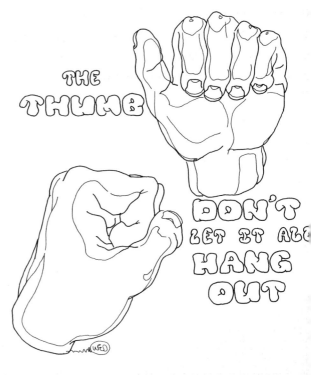

THE THUMB

DON'T LET IT ALL HANG OUT

Figure 3-Q: Thumb folded into and over fist

ski pole leverage forcing the thumb away from the body during an awkward fall. Skiers have renamed their common injury—"skier's" thumb.

Why the name "gamekeeper's"? Rumor has it that during the Middle Ages, the "keepers-of-the-game" for the kings and queens all suffered from a common affliction—loose and wobbly thumbs. Their job description included breaking the neck of rabbits served at banquets for knights, damsels, and royalty. The gruesome task was terminally (and hopefully humanely) ended by one quick snapping movement. There must have been some tough and determined rabbits or ineffective game managers. Needless to say—the thumb took a beating. Assuming that worker's compensation benefits were nonexistent, I wonder what their alternate duties or retirement was like.

Moral of the story? Wrap and protect the thumb. Punch correctly with your hand in proper position. Newly created "thumbless" and thumb-attached competition boxing gloves have been marketed recently. With the thumb section sewn into the main portion of the glove—injuries have declined accordingly. Figure 3-R) Training gloves or bag gloves lack this feature. Isn't it satisfying to possess a concrete example of industry modifications that have improved safety in such a direct, documentable manner? Eye injury in competitive boxers likewise improved as the attached thumb wasn't hanging out to inadvertently poke into the eye. Product improvement EQUALS improved safety! The martial arts industry desperately needs an unbiased, non-political product endorsement committee. Standards are non-existent and price absolutely controls the market. A positive model exists within the bicycle industry. Bicycle helmets are now required to meet minimum impact standards. Another positive role model has developed for amateur boxing. All competition gloves for U.S.A. Boxing must be certified by an assigned Safety Committee. On the

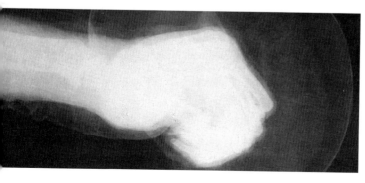

Figure 3-R: X-ray of hand in boxing glove. Notice incomplete, improperly positioned hand.

other hand, I am appalled by the oppressive medical-legal standards by which American football helmets are scrutinized by a few greedy plaintiffs. Hopefully, the martial arts industry will be level-headed in mandating useful, realistic standards.

SUMMARY OF FINGER INJURY TREATMENT

A few comments about common finger joint sprains will establish some basic guidelines for treatment.

1. Just as in any other joint—a sprain (of any severity) is a tearing of ligaments and capsular structures. These structures may be overpowered by any variety or combination of pulls, bends, twists, or compression forces.

2. Ice a swollen joint. Don't dip your entire hand into the pot. The ends of digits are very sensitive and it is not worth the pain. Simply use several ice cubes in a sandwich baggie to isolate the spot. (Sorry to be repetitious, but forget heat. Stick with ice for as many days as it takes to defeat the initial swelling, pain, feeling of "heat.") Limit ice sessions to about 10 to 15 minutes each. Utilize many frequent sessions during the day.

3. Apply a splint to any finger requiring rest. It is more practical for the splint to sit on the top (not palm side) of your finger. This position allows some tactile and gripping function for that fingertip. It is less cumbersome. (Figure 3-S and Figure 3-T)

4. After the acute need to splint your sprained finger (about 3 to 7 days) begin BUDDY TAPING. Use narrow ½-inch tape and encircle the adjacent digit in 2 spots. Choose areas that don't necessarily restrict the bending of your joints. If your long or ring finger

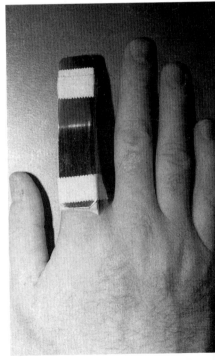

Figure 3-S: Appropriate method of splinting — top view

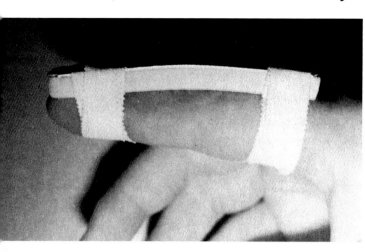

Figure 3-T: Appropriate method of splinting — side view

is injured, use the uninjured long or ring finger for splinting. In this configuration, the width of your grip is unhampered so that sports activities will be less impaired. (Figure 3-U and Figure 3-V)

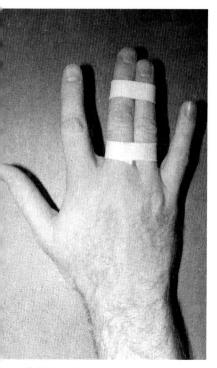

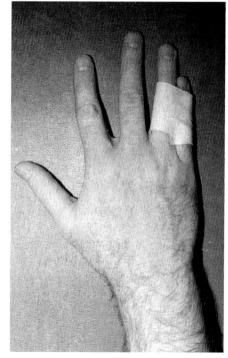

gure 3-U: Buddy taping — correct proce-
re

Figure 3-V: Buddy taping — incorrect procedure

5. BUDDY TAPING accomplishes 2 purposes:
   A. The injured digit is splinted and protected by its adjacent "buddy."
   B. Increasing and improving range of motion remains enhanced by its "good buddy" pulling along the injured "teammate." Conveniently, the injured joint is only urged into flexion-extension directions and not subjected to harmful twists and turns. A more rapid recovery is promoted. Your volunteer finger serves as a "physical therapist."
6. CAUTION: If you notice a deformity other than swelling in your finger visit a sportsmedicine physician. If your finger remains in some flexion with an inability to fully extend—see your doctor. If you suspect a fracture—see your doctor.

WRIST

"Durable Tim" was one tough cookie. He represented training intensity as a martial artist and volunteered unfailingly to be demonstrated upon for any throw, submission hold, or new technique. Mentally tough—always up and ready. Could he ever wail on a heavy bag! NO MERCY—grueling workouts.

Tim (with whom I have trained at times) came to my sportsmedicine clinic with a complaint that his wrist had been "achy" for several months but was now restricting the quality and intensity of his workouts. In fact—it even ached each following day in his duties as an electrician. My physical exam demonstrated some limitation in his extremes of movement as I guided his wrist into full extension (wrist cocked upward) and into full flexion (wrist pointed downward). His x-rays demonstrated cystic abnormalities in several of the small wrist bones suggesting the early onset of wear and tear arthritis at his young age of 35. His insistence upon grueling macro

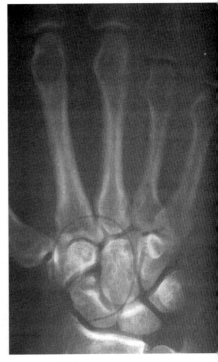

Figure 3-W: Wrist cystic abnormality

pounding sessions had sacrificed the longevity and painless function of his wrist joint. (Figure 3-W) Lesson? Remember what we said about **diversity** as the bedrock of the Boxergenics™ system? Let's learn the lessons taught to me by multiple patient-athletes. Rotate between many workout options. Don't get hung-up on a favorite technique or overload will occur.

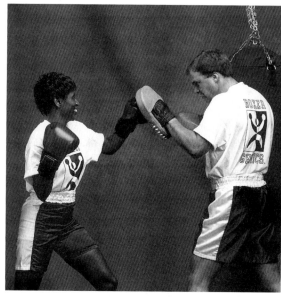

Figure 3-X: Focus pads

Punch the focus pad (Figure 3-X) or heavy bag (Figure 3-Y) with well placed straight-ahead blows. Crooked contact will force torque on your wrist and sprain the ligaments stabilizing top, bottom, or sides. These do require a prolonged rest period of several weeks if partially torn. If injured, there exists enough inherent flexibility in the science of Boxergenics™ to immediately transfer emphasis to shadow boxing or foot work to obtain a target heart rate and symmetric muscle toning. Utilization of the newly invented **"CORE-PAD"** training handwraps will vastly improve wrist stability. Incorporated straps assist in preventing extreme bending of your wrists. These handwraps vitally support wrists as importantly as they pad the hands.

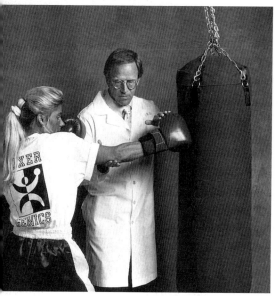

Figure 3-Y: Heavy bag

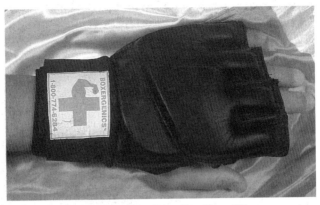

Figure 3-Z-1: Grappling Glove™

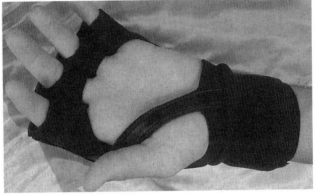

Figure 3-Z-2: Grappling Glove™

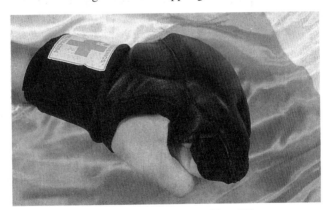

Figure 3-Z-3: Grappling Glove™

BOXERGENICS™

1-800-774-6284

The Grappling Glove recently added to protect the hands and decrease facial cuts of Ultimate Fighting and Battlecade Extreme Fighting contestants are pictured in Figures 3-Z-1, 3-Z-2, and 3-Z-3. They creatively benefit from a hybrid design, padding the striker's knuckles while the open-palm format does not disadvantage the grappler.

SCAPHOID FRACTURES

A peanut-shaped bone occupies the thumb side of your wrist and deserves its reputation as one of the most difficult-to-heal bones in the body. The wrist complexly exists as an organized puzzle of 8 separate bones, roughly divided as two rows bound together by ligaments. Each bone must accurately glide against its neighbor. Any malrotation or change in position will unbalance the flexion, extension, or rotation of your wrist. The scaphoid bone (formerly known as the navicular) happens to cross both rows and is subject to fracture across its mid-portion or waist. (Figure 3-AA) A tenuous blood supply creates problems in healing. Diagnosis

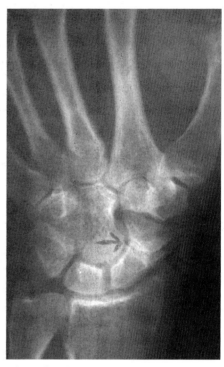

Figure 3-AA: X-ray of schaphoid fracture

must be achieved soon after injury so that early treatment can be initiated.

MECHANISM

An excessive, unbalanced load onto the wrist (such as generated in a poorly angled punch or a fall onto the hand) will crack the scaphoid.

Because the peanut-shaped scaphoid is so small, an early undisplaced crack may not show up on x-ray for several weeks. This places a challenge on yourself and your physician.

It often takes several weeks for bone to absorb around the fracture site and any sign of breakage to become visible. Your best chance for healing is dependent upon immediate immobilization of this injured bone. I have witnessed patients who, because of delay, required months of casting, surgical repair, electrical stimulation, or salvage procedures. Casts may be required for 4 or 5 months in difficult cases. OBTAIN EARLY TREATMENT IF YOU HAVE WRIST PAIN. If you have pain in your "snuff box" and sustained an injury of possible significance, splint your hand and wrist until x-rays have been initially obtained and remain negative for two weeks post injury. Tendon and ligament trauma to this same area of the wrist can often require weeks of treatment to resolve.

Chapter 4

Elbow

HYPEREXTENSION

Your elbow is a hinge-joint that moves from 0° (full extension) to about 140° (full flexion). (Figure 4-A) Usually one's arm is rarely forced by sports activity into a severely flexed or bent position. But, a boxer, martial artist, or wrestler may often find himself (herself) in a position where the elbow slams into forced straightening (extension). (Figure 4-A) This may occur to a wrestler when his arm is used as a pry and forced straighter than its normal stopping point. A boxer can miss a punch and the velocity of his effort overshoots the target causing a sudden snapping in the joint. Rarely, as an elbow extends at the conclusion of a punch, the backside of the elbow may be punched or blocked, suddenly forcing a hyperextension movement. Any one of these mechanisms can end in the same terrible sharp, burning pain. Coaches can also suffer injury, but more commonly to the medial (inside area) aspect of his elbow. Uncontrolled forces during focus pad drills can damage ligaments (Figure 4-B). Coaches should stay alert and punchers should control their force and direction of punches. Usually, nothing breaks and x-rays are normal. But, if enough joint bleeding occurs, fluid accumulation might show on the x-ray film. The resulting damage occurs within the ligaments as they are stretched beyond their normal elastic limits and microscopic tearing and bleeding results. The treatment? Never forget that highly effective mnemonic of athletic trainers—R.I.C.E.

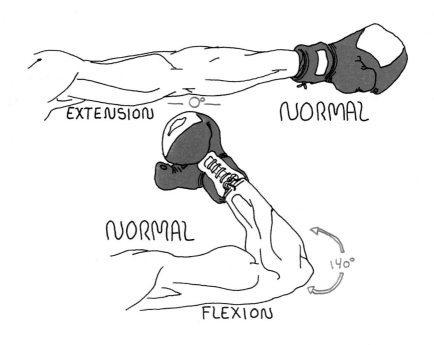

EXTENSION   NORMAL

NORMAL

140°

FLEXION

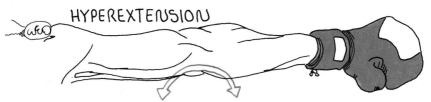

HYPEREXTENSION

ABNORMAL STRESS CAUSING INJURY

Figure 4-A: Elbow positions

— Rest
— Ice
— Compression
— Elevation

Rest the elbow in some flexion as it didn't appreciate being forced into over-extension. If it hurts enough—use a sling or visit your sportsmedicine specialist for a temporary splint.

Ice should be applied to both sides of the elbow. Either wrap the elbow with a large plastic bag of ice or use an elastic bandage to incorporate smaller bags around this joint. Sessions should last 10 to 15 minutes and there should be multiple sessions in one day.

Compression is not as useful for this type of injury since it is confined to an isolated area.

Elevation is likewise not quite as useful in an elbow as compared to injuries of the hand, wrist, foot, or knee.

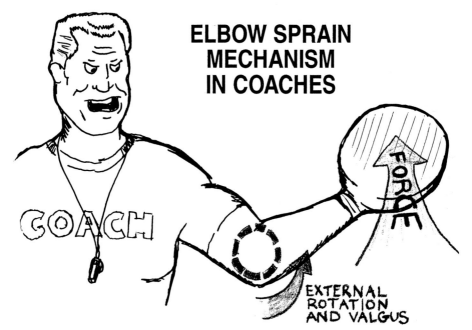

Figure 4-B: Elbow sprain mechanism in coaches

LONG MEMORY

Within several days start gentle movements so the elbow doesn't scar into unwanted stiffness. The body has a "long memory" so that the last activity it will let you perform is the unfortunate movement that initially hurt it. (Figure 4-C) Some workout movements can be cautiously performed within the increasingly painless arc.

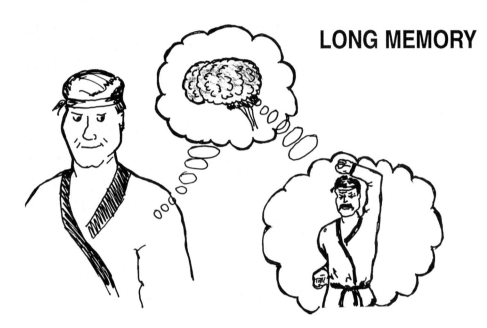

Figure 4-C: "Long memory" — The movement that injures an athlete is usually the last activity that they may resume.

As you are achieving full painless movement, a very handy taping technique must be learned. It is called "extension block" taping.

1. Anchor some strips of tape just above and just below the elbow

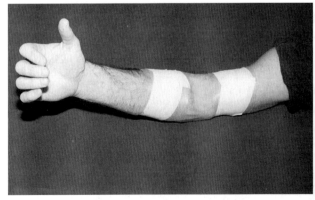

Figure 4-D: Extension block taping

joint. (Shave first if you don't want to be tortured removing the tape.) (Figure 4-D)

2. Keep the elbow slightly bent, maybe about 25°. Apply X-shaped layers of tape so they form a strut across the bend of your elbow. These "block" you from straightening fully. (Figure 4-E)

3. Lay a final layer over your initial anchoring tape to tie-in and secure the tape of step #2 from pulling loose. (Figure 4-F)

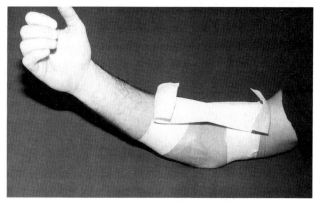

Figure 4-E: Extension block taping

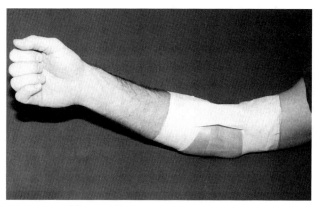

Figure 4-F: Extension block taping

Now you can punch without the fear of your arm over-straightening. Utilize this taping technique as long as the troublesome movement produces pain.

TENNIS ELBOW

Although not related to the act of punching, tendonitis on the lateral aspect (outside) of the elbow may occur as a training injury. Tennis elbow is most usually an overuse phenomenon and rarely occurs suddenly or from a direct blow or fall. Gripping an arnis (kali) stick, tennis racquet or golf club (Figure 4-G) can transmit excess stress and shock to the forearm muscle's tendon insertion onto the elbow. Study your own forearm. The outside (lateral aspect) has much less bulk than the medial (inside) musculature. Thus, excessively applied stress will more likely "pull" tendons laterally than medially. That's

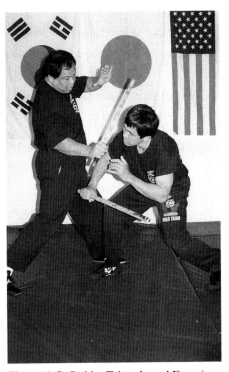

why the back hand stroke in tennis more commonly tears lateral (extensor) muscle insertions than the forehand stroke which predominantly loads the medial (flexor) surface.

What is the pathology if we peer into a microscope? A section of the tendon insertion has been torn and haphazard attempts at scar formation have formed. (Figure 4-H) Every time we tense this muscle, we pull against the abnormal cross-fibers within this little ball of scar. Normally, external forces exert internal forces that parallel the grain of well-organized tendon fibers. Pain is produced as we pull "against the grain."

Figure 4-G: Bobby Taboada and Francisco Gaerlan gripping arnis sticks

The lateral forearm muscles are especially tensed when we grip an object in a backhand direction. Eventually, in traumatized tendons even clenching the fist activates enough pressure for symptoms. Extending the wrist or fingers against resistance really creates problems. Weightlifters will notice that pushing movements are reasonably well tolerated but pulling movements most noticeably create symptoms.

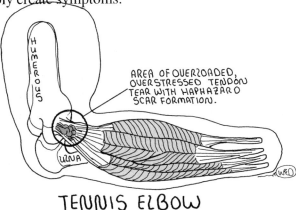

TENNIS ELBOW

Figure 4-H: Tennis elbow scar formation

TREATMENT

1. Identify the cause of each problem. Fix it! Were your training sessions with the arnis sticks too arduous? Did reverse curls with dumbbells aggravate it? Was pulling on the lat machine overloading your elbow? Should you give up tennis and golf and spend more time in safer sports like boxing and karate??? After all, this is called "tennis elbow."

2. Modify workout patterns so as not to anger the healing tissue. If you don't you will produce a chronic problem. Solve this one early and shorten your potential total down-time. For example:
   • Use arnis sticks in a forward swing only and not in backhand swings.
   • Perform push exercises such as presses rather than **pull** exercises such as chins and lat pull-downs.
   • Perform uppercut movements on the training bag rather than snapping out and fully "turning-over" your punches.
   • Generally palm-up activities are o.k., **palm facing downward** lifting activities are to be avoided.

3. Ice the injury.

4. Anti-inflammatories like Ibuprofen help only a little bit. They can never make up for improper forces or aggravating mechanical movements.

5. Conscientiously wear a tennis elbow splint when active, lifting, carrying objects, or working out. They probably work by broadening and dispersing the attachment forces over a more extensive surface area. They unload the injured tissue and absorb some of the stresses before they are directed into the area of tear. Don't wear this when inactive or sleeping.

6. Transverse massage or ice massage can be useful, especially when properly taught by a therapist or athletic trainer. (**NOTE: Fill a small paper dixie cup with water and freeze it. Peel away some of the rim. Allow the ice surface to melt down so as not to be abrasive. Now perform the massage with the cup, gaining the benefits of massage plus ice**).

7. Visit a physical therapist or trainer for galvanic stim, ultrasound, or cortisone iontophoresis treatments.

8. Initiate a stretch and strength program for the forearm muscles when you have improved enough to shake hands comfortably. Can you imagine what a curse tennis elbow would be to a campaigning politician? An easy, convenient method for strengthening the extensor muscles is as simple as a rubber band around the fingers. Carry it in your pocket for convenient rehab sessions all day. (Figure 4-I)

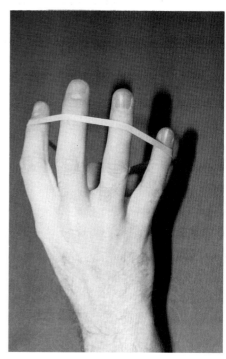

Figure 4-I: Rubber band exercises for rehab of extensor muscles/forearm

9. A judicious injection of cortisone by a sports physician can result in a progressive and permanent cure. I do perform these with the **intention** of fixing the problem, not just masking it, but detailing an explanation that recurrence is common. The patient must understand this reasoning. A properly applied injection can cure the problem if the patient:

   A. Ceases or modifies the offending activity.

   B. Allows the tissue to heal.

   C. Slowly strengthens and stretches the injured muscle units.

   D. Has luck on his side.

   One must realize that the "shot" is not the cure, but simply quiets down the irritation and **initiates** the start of the healing process that takes about **6 weeks.**

10. Resistant cases may need up to 3 shots, spread out over many weeks. I rarely repeat this shot before 4 weeks have passed. I am hopeful that I have increased the circulation to the affected area and that the body can now complete its healing cycle of events.

Generally, three shots spread-out over time are the maximum amount that I recommend. If progress is occurring, a fourth shot is occasionally acceptable. But, if three shots haven't worked, ten shots won't do it either. In summary, **"3 strikes and you're out!"**.

My technique of injection involves using a small needle (no larger than 25 gauge). A sterile skin prep with Betadine and sterile gloves are used. Sterile technique must be scrupulously observed. The skin is desensitized by ethyl chloride spray.

An injection of 1cc (¼%) Marcaine, 1cc (1%) Xylocaine, and ½cc to 1cc of Cortisone is utilized. Usually a total of 3cc is injected into the site of maximum tenderness and pathologically injured tissue. The elbow is positioned at a bend of approximately 70° to 90°. Once under the skin, I consider it important to perform multiple punctures (8 to 12) to the area of the poor tissue in order to elicit a healing response. I am trying to "rev up" a "stalled out" sequence of events that returns a fresh blood supply to the area while providing relief of discomfort. Why perforate the injured tissue? One of my most respected, but now deceased, mentors Dr. George Rovere lucidly and simplistically explained it to me this way … "If you want to promote healing, make the tissue think it's injured." We thus precipitate the cascade of physiologic events that the body can miraculously organize in order to heal.

11. If all conservative treatment has, in good conscience, been followed and three shots have failed, surgery is indicated.

GOLFER'S ELBOW

The pathology and treatment options for tendonitis on the medial aspect are quite similar to those of tennis elbow. Because a larger muscle mass exists on the flexor surface of the forearm, healing is slower.

In daily activity and exercises, the **palm-up** position is actively loading the injured tissue and should be avoided. A **palm-down** grip is a preferred position which lessens the load on the injured flexor muscle mass. Tennis elbow splints can help.

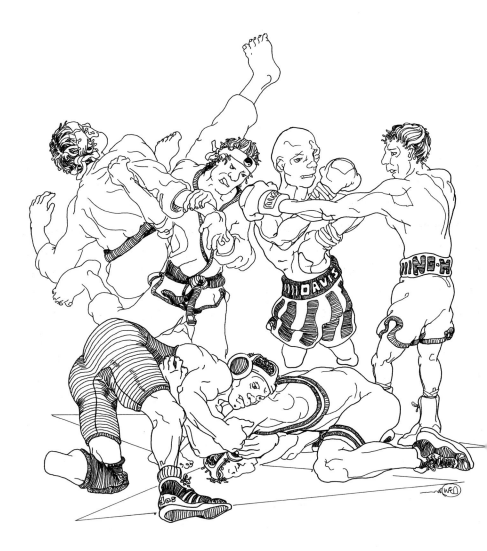

Chapter 5

Shoulder

The shoulder is a very complex joint and we, as sportsmedicine scientists, agree that our understanding of the functional anatomy (and things that can go wrong with the anatomy) falls about 10 years short of what we have learned about the knee. The highly supple shoulder isn't as simple a concept to grasp as the single-plane hinged-joint elbow. One should not view this mechanical complex as just "one big shoulder joint." The proper approach demands viewing the shoulder, with its individualized components, as one might understand the complex engine of a car. The average car owner doesn't return his car to the repair shop simply generalizing that "it's broken—fix it." To expect a reasonable effort at repair, a more selective summary of pertinent problems must be stated. Just because one directs repair efforts toward a faulty fan belt, does not guarantee that valves, radiator, and distributor do not need attention or investigation. Fortunately, we can likewise "compartmentalize" the shoulder into its various functioning units. By examining each area and potentially performing tests or injections to one area at a time, we can often sort out which portion of the shoulder initiates problems. Thus, in evaluating the shoulder, one must realize that we should be comprehensively inspecting many separate components of shoulder anatomy by various testing procedures.

UNDERSTANDING THE BIOMECHANICS

We might relate the shoulder to a ball and socket, but with a very shallow socket. See photo of normal shoulder joint obtained during arthroscopic surgery. This shows the normal slightly concave "socket" on the left and the smooth rounded humeral head "ball" on the right. (Figure 5-A) Therefore, it can travel through a great carefree arc, but there is a price to pay for all of that freedom of movement—stability. Since the component bones don't encompass and cradle this joint—ligaments and tendons must "shoulder" this responsibility. Great analogy—huh! We expect a lot from our shoulder during athletic feats and tremendous power (strength X speed) can be generated.

Scientists have likened the mechanics of throwing a pitch to an "explosion." Researchers have gathered extensive functional knowledge from studying slow speed cinematography of pitchers. When you

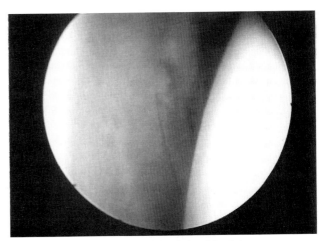

Figure 5-A: Normal shoulder joint

stop and think about it, most of our sports movements rely upon similar basic actions. Doesn't our arm go through many of the same positions as we "throw" a tennis racquet to hit a ball, "throw" a barbell as we perform a bench press, "throw" our hand into the water as we swim, "throw" a punch as we hit the bag? As most of the explosive action is directed **forward,** the muscles and tendons in the front of your shoulder tend to become dominantly strong and contracted, while the smaller structures at the back of the shoulder become sacrificed to weakness and overstretch. We summarize the problem as "Mercedes muscles up front and Volkswagen muscles in the rear." (Figure 5-B)

ROTATOR CUFF

The often referred to but poorly understood "rotator cuff" is derived from a group of four companion muscles that cover and anchor the humeral head—the ball portion of this "ball and socket" joint. They steer and direct the humeral head to remain centered as our arm is traveling through all of those crazy,

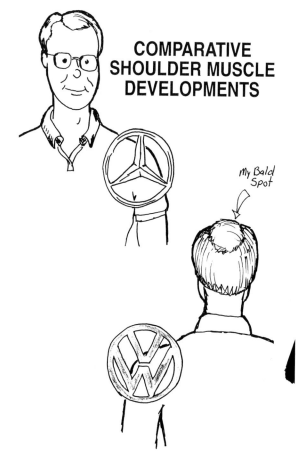

COMPARATIVE SHOULDER MUSCLE DEVELOPMENTS

My Bald Spot

Figure 5-B: Comparative shoulder muscle development. Don't forget the posterior shoulder muscles during your workouts. Dr. Estwanik advises one set of posterior rotator cuff exercises for every set of bench presses.

demanding sports motions. Good tone and balance of the rotator cuff assure a smooth arc, maintaining the joint's "instant-center." This arrangement prevents violent erratic jumping-about within our joint as the large exterior muscles exert their powerful effects, i.e., punching, throwing, bench pressing. Most strength training efforts are directed towards and absorbed by our larger muscle groups (like the traps, lats, deltoids, etc.) and the rotator cuff group can unknowingly be undertrained and weak unless specifically targeted by very specific exercises. This explains why a lightning-fast pitcher can still be flirting with the danger of a downhill course initiated by an unsupportive and weak cuff.

The rotator cuff group (subscapularis, supraspinatus, infraspinatus, teres minor muscles) lives in a rather confined space between the humeral head and the overlying acromion. Clearance space is critical for painless non-pinched function. (Figure 5-C) Simply think in terms of a family living within a confined room in a house. They need enough "elbow room" (or in this case "shoulder room") to safely and comfortably move about. If their space becomes confined, those living in that area will become bruised and injured.

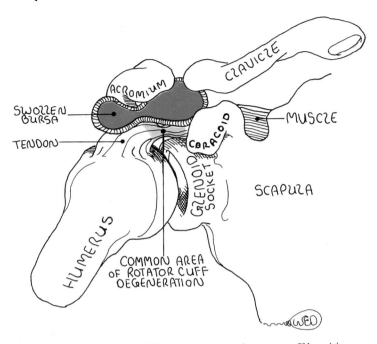

Figure 5-C: Rotator cuff impingement and rotator cuff bursitis

The rotator cuff is prone to injury and degeneration because of its intrinsic confinement between two bony layers—the humeral head on the floor and the acromion forming the ceiling. As we raise our arm overhead, as required for most sports activities, the size of our "room" is narrowed and compromised. Those who are fortunately born with a more spacious room will intrinsically escape injury by a greater margin of error. Those born with a downward sloping acromion are set-up for tendonitis, bursitis, impingement, and rotator cuff tears. The supraspinatus tendon is the area most likely to get smashed in overhead activities—it is the "critical zone." Doctors have been able to describe x-ray classification of acromions into types based upon their shape and likelihood of causing problems.

How do you suspect a problem? The classical presenting conditions of tendonitis, bursitis, and impingement are quite similar and related. These diagnoses are inter-related and somewhat interchangeable. If you have one problem, you are placed in the same set of circumstances for sustaining the other diagnoses.

The subacromial bursa serves as a lubricated balloon between your rotator cuff and its overlying bony ceiling, the acromion. Anything that pinches the bursa will cause it to become angry, swollen, thick, and produce irritation fluid instead of the slick motor oil that functions for lubrication. Irritation of this bursa is called rotator cuff **bursitis.** Repeated activities that pinch tissues can cause bursitis and inflammation of the rotator cuff tendon components. This can finally culminate in a **rotator cuff tear**—the end-stage fatigue and fraying of that sandwiched tendon layer. Grinding and pain in your shoulder from repetitive rotational sports movements may point the finger of blame to any of the conditions mentioned: tendonitis, bursitis, and impingement.

SUBLUXATIONS/DISLOCATIONS

Watch out for a shoulder that feels like it is "slipping" out of socket associated with popping and aching. A sensation of slipping or instability could harbor the beginnings of a very rough and rocky journey to a surgical stabization (tightening) procedure. The rather shallow shoulder joint provides a marvelous arc of motion but sacrifices inherent stability to accomplish the job. As compared to the hip joint which is very stable but limiting in the final positions that we can place our foot, the shoulder joint has given us plenty of movement—sometimes too much. The classic mechanism of injury occurs when the arm is forced overhead—both too far from the shoulder (abduction) and too far behind the head (external rotation). (Figure 5-D, 5-E, 5-F) A martial artist can "slip" into problems if her arm arm gets over-extended during a high block. Any wrestler shoots into the "at-risk" position as his arm is outstretched during take down or switching maneuvers. These classically "bad news" positions are rare for a boxer but he swings into problems with a "missed" punch. The speeding arm misses the target and "taken-by-surprise" muscles don't have time to react in a deceleration mode—the arm just "keeps on truckin'," stretching the critically necessary ligaments located at the front of the shoulder. Coaches are also at risk for the same forces that abnormally stress a shoulder joint. Any mechanism that forces a shoulder joint past its normal stopping point places the athlete or coach at risk. Remain alert and in control during training sessions. (Figure 5-G)

An explanation and clarification of medical terms may help you avoid the confusion that I routinely anticipate in patients/athletes. The term SUBLUXATION describes a "partial" dislocation. The unstable shoulder never fully

MECHANISM OF SHOULDER DISLOCATION-SUBLUXATION

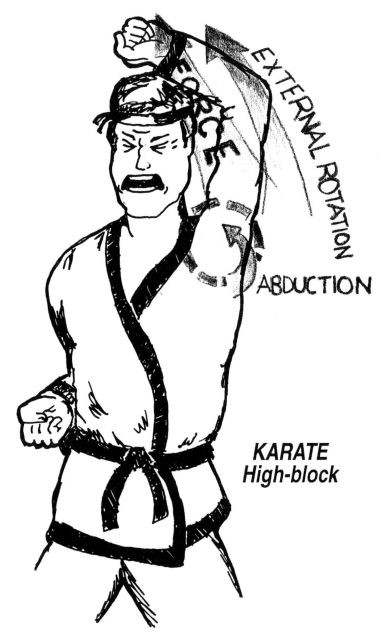

Figure 5-D: Shoulder dislocation/subluxation (karate)

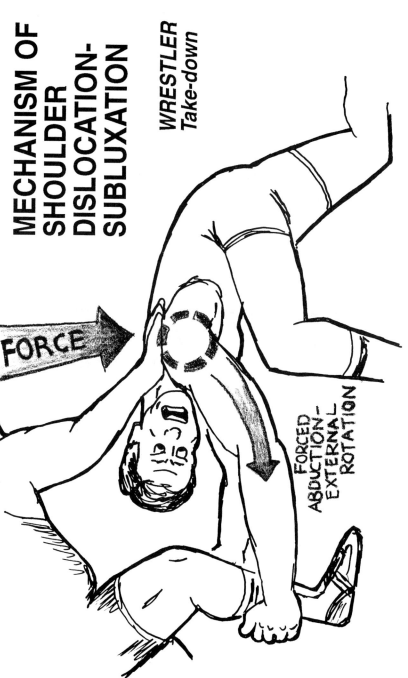

Figure 5-E: Shoulder dislocation/subluxation (wrestler)

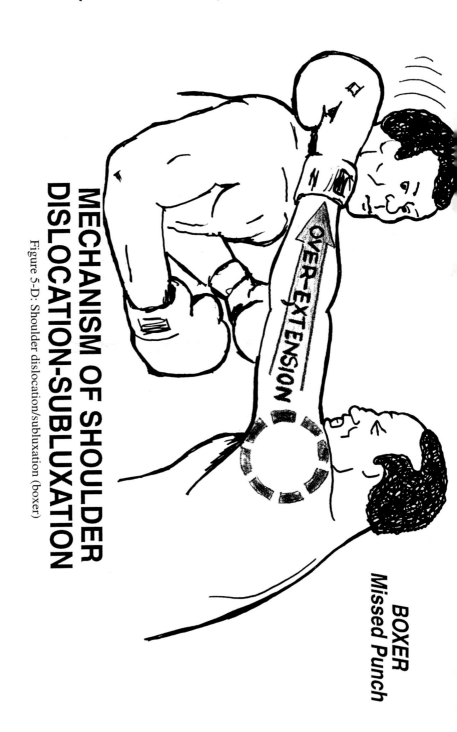

MECHANISM OF SHOULDER
DISLOCATION-SUBLUXATION

Figure 5-D: Shoulder dislocation/subluxation (boxer)

OVER-EXTENSION

BOXER
Missed Punch

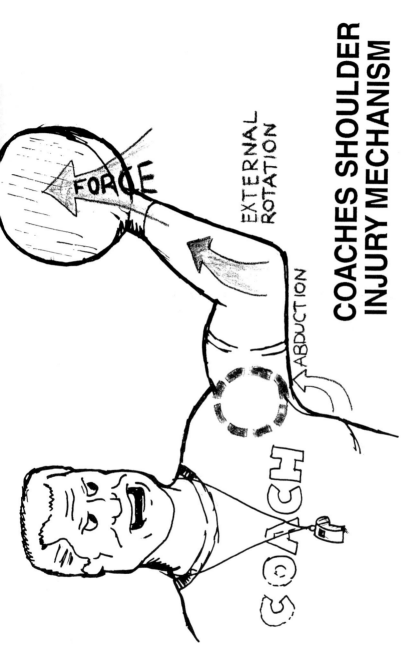

Figure 5-G: Mechanism that forces a shoulder past its normal stopping point

falls out of the socket and the sensation of a slip is more instantaneous and transient. It never jumps fully out of place and never requires someone to reduce it (pull it back in place) as often occurs in a DISLOCATION.

Subluxations may be just as functionally limiting as dislocations since these "partial dislocations" may occur many times a day and force one to cease a sport or completely avoid particular movements within a sport. As the same tissues are torn in each condition, the difference arises mainly in the degree of damage.

TREATMENT FOR SUBLUXATIONS/DISLOCATIONS

Unless treated aggressively by strict immobilization in a sling for 3 - 6 weeks, the tissues will heal in a stretched-out position. The "golden period" for the tissues to heal back-in-place peaks when the bleeding and trauma are fresh and the engines of repair are revving. The initial treatment of dislocating and subluxing shoulders has been controversially and classically handled in a rather cavalier manner. That is, a sling for a few days, minor toning exercises, then gradual return to activity. Torn ligaments cannot and do not heal under these conditions by the statistical fact that should a teenager dislocate his shoulder—he stands an 80% chance that this will recur until major surgery is performed. Doctors have never advocated treatment for corresponding knee ligament tear in such a casual manner! Therapy exercises can help to a certain extent, but only to a point. Exercise strengthens muscle, but the pathology in a dislocating shoulder is not occurring at the muscle layer. Deep capsular tissues primarily are ruptured loose in a dislocation and don't respond to exercising.

The final corrective treatment for a repetitive and repeatedly dislocating shoulder (fully pops out of socket) and a more subtle subluxing shoulder (partially slips out) is quite similar. The same structures are injured and these same structures must be stabilized, reconnected, and shortened. Imagine that you had too much "blousiness" in the front seams of your dressy white shirt. Imagine that the seams had been torn. A surgeon or seamstress would, by similar paths (one sterile and the other less so), take a tuck and re-anchor the excess material. Generally the surgeon has had to accomplish this 96% successful task by open surgery but recent advances in arthroscopic surgery are modifying the options. Some scope techniques allow the surgeon to utilize laser tool to "shrink wrap" the stretched tissues in less severe cases.

AC (ACROMIOCLAVICULAR) JOINT INJURY

There is a little joint sitting atop the shoulder that is sometimes forgotten or confused with its big brother, the glenohumeral joint. Athletes often confuse their respective location of injuries.

ACUTE INJURY

An injury which distorts the AC joint complex and causes deformity is termed a SEPARA-TION. (Figure 5-H) Shoulder dislocations have been thoroughly discussed in prior sections. AC joint injury usually occurs by way of a direct fall onto the point of the shoulder. The arm itself is usually not a factor in the sequence of events and is usually tucked safely aside the chest. In fact, the top of the shoulder absorbs too much

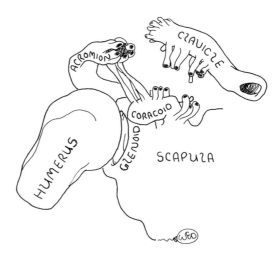

A.C. JOINT SUBLUXATION

Figure 5-H: AC joint subluxation

of the force at the time of impact. The jiu-jitsu competitor or wrestler if forcefully landing onto the shoulder might force the shoulder and arm downward away from the clavicle. His body roll, which usually would dissipate the force of falling, would not have been properly utilized to distribute the landing forces.

The classic deformity is a large bump atop the shoulder. Pain and temporary inability to lift the shoulder are immediate. Severity is graded as small 1°), medium (2°), large (3°), and severe (4°). Get an x-ray for confirmation f diagnosis and severity grading!

TREATMENT

A. 1° sprains can be treated very conservatively. Ice, a sling for a few days, and anti-inflammatories will suffice. Start early movement and gradual strengthening. A small bump may persist. An actual compression of the joint by a sideways-force during the injury could lead to future arthritis of the joint.

B. 2° injuries show a greater bump or prominence of the clavicle (collar bone). More ligaments were torn and more pain results. You may have problems sleeping at night for several days. A simple sling won't reduce the injury but a special AC sling can vastly improve the distortion and reduce the separation to a more minor deformity. An AC sling is useful for grades II and III but is a very uncomfortable apparatus that requires physician monitoring weekly. It can definitely work and save one surgery or deformity. These slings must be worn constantly for three to six weeks. Complications can include skin problems and stiffness.

C. 3° separations need either the AC splint or acceptance of a rather obvious bump. Occasionally surgery is optional for a very athletic individual or one who won't tolerate being confined in the sling. One must even sleep semi-sitting for the sling to work. The weight of the arm hanging down in the sling actually decreases and improves the separation.

D. Huge 4° separations are severe and need surgery.

CHRONIC INJURY

Those heavily involved in weight training and specifically the "bench press" can develop pressure-compression related inflammation and degeneration of the AC joint. A constant ache, pain in this joint when sleeping on your side, and soreness after exercise are common complaints. Often, a slight prominence and soreness to touch cause a patient to seek help. A weightlifter undoubtedly sees his bench press abilities go downhill. Highly repetitive activities that produce great forces on the shoulder such as training with kali sticks or months of punching a heavy bag with continued full force can wear this joint. An x-ray will demonstrate narrowing of the AC joint space and actual resorption, deformity, and cystic formations within the distal collar bone. (Figure 5-I)

A well respected high school basketball coach, Kevin, came to my office with continuous aching on the top of each shoulder. He loved weight training as an exercise form and was disappointed that this pain had dropped his bench press from 250 pounds down to a frustrating 135 pound level. He also taught physical education and was accurate in his lifting technique and dedicated to fitness. I could find no fault in his technique and reasoned that simple over load at 40 years old was the only explanation. I injected cortisone into each

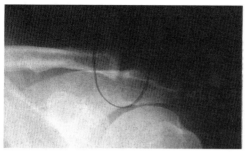

Figure 5-I: X-ray of worn AC joint (pre-op)

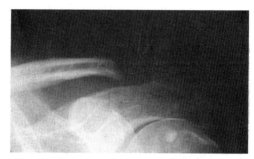

Figure 5-J: X-ray of post-op AC joint excision

AC joint and he did improve for several months. A slow decline again brought him back to the clinic for a second trial of injections. He did follow instructions to decrease his bench press workouts and push-up program. He could never regain a pain-free exercise program nor sustain his upper body strength levels. Surgery was requested and I appropriately counseled him in his options (which were few).

SURGERY (Figure 5-J)

The surgery essentially consists of excising (removing) the end 1cm to 1½cm of the clavicle. Thus, there remains no joint surface to rub, become arthritic, or ache. The very logical question that I would anticipate your asking is—will this surgery weaken my shoulder? Not long ago, in my private practice, a patient arrived for treatment of an ankle injury. He did look familiar and review of his chart identified him as having AC joint surgery five years ago. Of course I questioned him as to his level of comfort and function. He reported no pain and proudly announced that he currently bench pressed within five pounds of his personal record, despite being five years older. This operation once performed cannot be undone or reversed. One has to be sure that the pertinent complaints originate very specifically from this location. I always test my patients with several xylocaine and cortisone injections over several months. If there is a firm relationship then one can be clear of conscience to recommend surgery. I recently treated a new patient, who despite the history of a recent AC joint excision, continued to experience his same pre-op pain, if not a worsened condition. Upon further history, his former surgeon had never injected a "test dose" into this joint before permanent excision. Patients and doctors must strive to be conservative in their expectations, demands, and actions. Always, always go one-step-at-a-time!

EXAMINATION TECHNIQUES

How should you be evaluated? First of all, organize your complaints and have a "gut feel" whether the symptoms stem from your shoulder in the first place. Shoulder pain can be rather non-specific and tricky. So much so that the shoulder has been labeled "the great masquerader." Angina (chest pain) certainly has been recognized to radiate into the shoulder and commonly down into the left arm. Gall bladder attacks, injured lungs, lung tumors, and ruptured discs in the neck all can add to the confusion. I once cared for a young airline pilot who sought help for an ache in his shoulder. X-rays revealed a large cyst eroding the end of his collarbone that proved to be a metastatic lesion from lung cancer. He was a cigarette smoker!

Providing information on how you got injured can accelerate your doctor's focus just like your directing the auto mechanic to the probable corner of your engine hiding the annoying squeak. The mechanic might, otherwise, have to circle the block for hours if left in the dark by your lack of guidance. Personally, my automobile squeaks miraculously disappear as if the nose of my car smells the driveway of the dealership. This recall can be enhanced in patients if guiding questions are utilized by your sports specialist. Many weightlifters who aggressively train in the bench press will develop biceps tendonitis or AC joint inflammation. Without hesitation, we transfer the recalcitrant shoulder over to physical therapy for a bench press workout. I'll then examine the patient soon after his session with the enhanced ability of the patient to accurately point out "the spot" and allow us to hear or feel the rub or squeak. Commonly, runners will be instructed to wear their running gear so that a jog in the vicinity of the office will "freshen" the leg symptoms. If you are "into" your sport, you as an athlete can breakdown that punch or kick into its component parts and explain what specific aspect magnifies the pain. Is it a twist? Is it during acceleration or deceleration? Is it with the elbow flexed or extended? Is your arm overhead, etc., etc.?

Now for the examination! Men remove your shirt and women wear a bathing suit top. Your sports physician must evaluate you as a whole person before he/she takes a microscope to your shoulder. Only by comparing left to right will a sense of symmetry and balance be evident. Your deltoid muscle should display the same roundness on left as right. Have the doctor view you from the backside. Those of us in sportsmedicine are only now realizing the vast importance and interplay of muscles connecting to and stabilizing our scapula (wing bone). Dr. Ben Kibler of Lexington, Kentucky who supervises many elite tennis players, has expounded upon the large consequences of subtle weaknesses. A wing bone that flairs outward or fails to symmetrically rotate as one raises their arms to the front or to the sides means trouble. An unstable base of support for the shoulder joint improperly distributes forces placed on joint structures: tendons, ligaments, muscles, and joint surfaces. A house built upon a mushy foundation will eventually develop nail pops, squeaky floors, and cracking plaster. This explains why current, progressive rehab programs always include exercises to address weakened scapular muscles.

EXAMINATION SUGGESTIONS FOR THOROUGHNESS

1. Face toward your doctor with arms at your sides. Lift your arms forward, overhead, and to the side. Let him observe.

2. Face away from your doctor and repeat those movements.

3. If you notice grinding or noises, the physician should place his hand upon that area and request that you actively move your limb. He will also ask you to relax and will guide your shoulder passively through those same areas of movement.

4. Direct palpation of your SC (sternoclavicular) joint, AC (acromioclavicular) joint, collar bone, biceps tendon area, rotator cuff attachment area, and posterior shoulder area will ensure thoroughness.

5. By assuming the Estwanik "prone and propped" position, (Figure 5-K),

those deeply hidden and elusive focuses of tendonitis (levator scapulae syndrome) will rotate more superficially. If indicated, this structure should be injected only while in this "safe" position. (Figure 5-L)

6. Your arm will be brought fully across your chest and fully overhead in forward flexion to intentionally demonstrate a "pinch" if rotator cuff impingement is the culprit.

7. Your arm will intentionally be brought into full abduction and external rotation as if putting your hand up behind the back of your head. This is the vulnerable "at risk" position that causes 90% of dislocations or subluxations (partial dislocations). Any nervousness, ranging from apprehension to panic, while assuming this posturing lends strong suspicion of an unstable shoulder. Other maneuvers may be utilized.

8. Strength testing of the muscles in the shoulder and shoulder girdle can assist in prescribing a customized rehabilitation program.

9. Normal circulation and sensation of your entire arm and hand should be confirmed to rule out thoracic outlet syndrome.

10. Move your neck around. Pinched nerves in the neck can often refer pain towards the shoulder and fool you into suspecting an injury of shoulder origin rather than a radiation towards the shoulder.

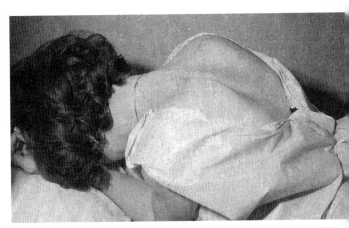

Figure 5-K: Estwanik "prone and propped" position suggested during each shoulder exam

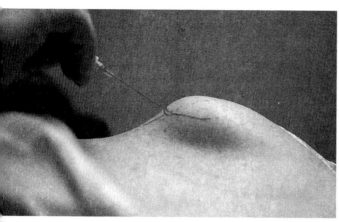

Figure 5-L: Injection of levator scapulae while in Estwanik "prone and propped" position

HINTS

In training, the Boxergenics™ system (Figure 5-M) allows you the opporunity to exercise and tone the shoulder from different angles to prevent repettive injury. Punch high, punch medium, punch low. Vary it! The jab, straight punch, hook, and uppercut each have characteristic angles from which we challenge the shoulder structures. Don't always aim or punch at eye level. Vary your aim from eye level to mid-abdomen. Utilize that versatility inherent in his art. Before and after class, warm-up and stretch your shoulder thoroughy. Should a shoulder problem develop in any sporting activity, consult a physcal therapist or sportsmedicine specialist early so that you can be taught a successful group of exercises proven very effective for the "throwing" athlete. Do this to avoid future shoulder surgery. (Just for fun, quickly say **shoulder urgery** five times). Avid tennis players and baseball pitchers, by the nature f their sports, develop asymmetrically. Their sports make them lopsided, not nly from front-to-back but from dominant to non-dominant limb. We have o problem documenting the right-left distortions caused by their asymmetic training and performance techniques. One simply has to measure the left ersus right forearm and upper arm girth of tennis players to reveal the problem. I have witnessed x-rays of the contrasting **humerus** bones (upper arm ones) of throwers and fail to find the left versus right differences one bit unny. The bones in the dominant arm are actually and visibly hypertrophied increased in size), just as are the muscles. Boxing fitness training gives you

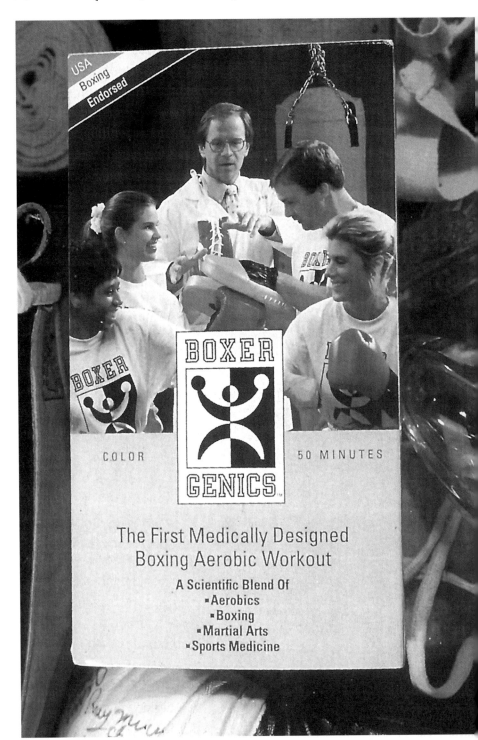

Figure 5-M: Boxergenics™ video cover

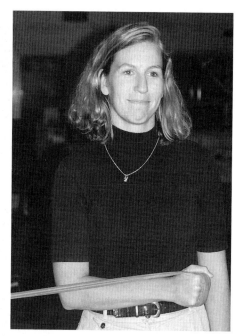

Figure 5-N: Rehab exercises for rotator cuff — Internal rotation using resistive band

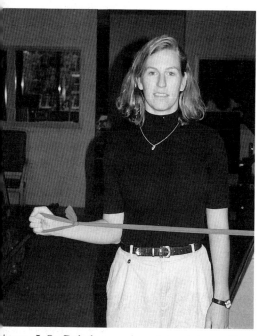

Figure 5-O: Rehab exercises for rotator cuff — External rotation using resistive band

the distinct advantage of incorporating symmetric goal-oriented techniques for both left and right application.

Over the past ten years, great advances in physical therapy have significantly prolonged the careers of many upper-body athletes (throwers, swimmers, racquet sports). Boxers and martial artists, in my opinion, remain in the Dark Ages. Recent strength testing of elite boxers in training camp substantiates unbelievably poor upper body development. Simply training in your sport doesn't provide that baseline development necessary for maximum strength, power, endurance, and injury prevention. Modern swimmers can't just swim! Modern boxers can't just box! Carefully study and perform the following injury preventing exercises to become a better athlete and prolong your career! These exercises in addition to routine weight training will protect all areas of the rotator cuff. (Figures 5-N, 5-O, 5-P, 5-Q, 5-R)

Routine weight lifting exercises fail to properly isolate the

POSTERIOR ROTATOR CUFF which is critically necessary to decelerate the arm after a punch is thrown. Routinely use these exercises as a part of your training program.

PREVENTION HINTS

1. Boxers and martial artists—Don't wail away on the heavy bag workout after workout. Vary your routine.

2. Bench pressers—If you sense a pattern developing, change your routine and lighten-up! Include posterior shoulder exercises.

3. Those with prior AC separations—Learn which exercises and sports tend to irritate the shoulder.

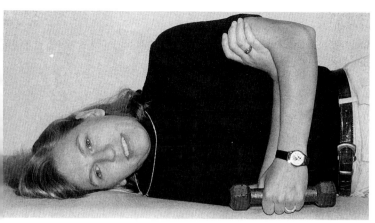

Figure 5-P: Rehab exercises for rotator cuff — Strengthening starting position using dumbbell

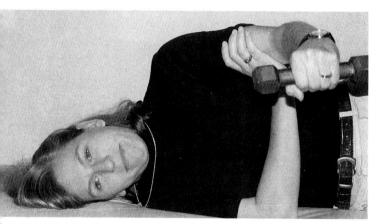

Figure 5-Q: Rehab exercises for rotator cuff — Strengthening ending position using dumbbell

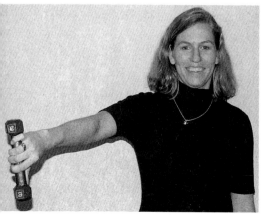

Figure 5-R: Rehab exercises for rotator cuff (supraspinatus) — "Empty can" strengthening

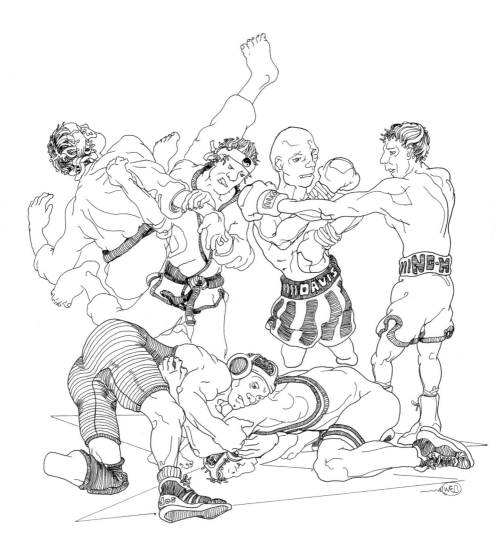

Chapter 6

Chest Injury

S killed punchers and kickers certainly should and do focus aggressive attention to the opponent's "body" (torso) for many reasons.

1. **The chest-thorax provides a large effective target area** for an opponent. Boxing coaches do discourage their athletes from "head hunting," i.e., placing too much emphasis on punching an opponent's head instead of aiming shots to the "body." Boxing gym wisdom proclaims "work the body and the head will follow." Translated into civilized civilian terms this means that repeated blows to the abdomen and ribcage will weaken an opponent. As he increasingly tucks-in elbows to shield his now tender ribs, the protective defense of his head and his ability to snap-out crisp punches will diminish. Don't underestimate a good solid blow to the torso. I have witnessed many a clean shot to the ribs or abdomen suddenly drop a boxer to the mat and end a bout. You don't have to knock-out an adversary or sporting opponent to triumph.

2. **Chances of injuring a hand or foot** are lessened as an offensive maneuver is directed to the more forgiving trunk region.

   In caring for competitors during the Ultimate Fighting Championships, I graphically witnessed how rock-hard the skull has been designed and how effectively it may traumatize the assaulting hand. There may be a "handsome" price to pay when the fist contacts the vault-like human skull.

One of the spectacular highlights of the UFC involved Keith Hackney, a Kempo fighter from Chicago. This 6'1", 215 pound fighter dramatically defeated a 6'9", 400 pound Sumo fighter with repeated punches to the back of the head once Keith was able to topple this imposing giant. Despite triumphing, brave Keith was physically unable to advance in the tournament because his hands were mincemeat. No fractures were sustained, as confirmed by follow-up x-rays, but the soft tissue damage made his grotesquely swollen hands resemble uncooked sausage. The point of the story being—the "body" is much softer than the skull. Your hands will pay a penalty for landing head blows. Not so on the body.

3. **The chest-abdomen exists as an easier to find target** than the elusive head. Whether the frontal plane of the chest-abdomen area or head is hit, a valid amateur boxing point is scored. USA Boxing's scoring philosophy awards no greater points for a head blow than for a cleanly scoring strike to the body. "Body" means the surface area below the neck and above the groin. In formal amateur bouts only strikes to the "frontal" plane are scoreable. In a street fight, effective punishments to the kidney area or posterior ribs constitute effective reality.

During aspects of my seven year limited exposure to law enforcement training—firearms instructors incessantly lectured about the effectiveness of grouping shots to the "center-of-mass." Purposely aiming at a criminal's head versus the much larger chest-abdomen constitutes a great error in judgment and a foolhardy practice that can result in a dead police officer. Aim for the center-of-mass. That's why police silhouette targets award as many points to the "center-of-mass" as the diminutive head area. I have overheard many boxing coaches preach the wisdom of aiming a respectful percentage of punches to this center-of-mass rather than an elusive bobbing head. Should a boxer duck—bingo—the jackpot is struck anyway.

For all of these reasons, the ribcage suffers an accumulated array of insults, most being temporary, minor, and fleeting. One must understand a confusing and not well known fact of the ribcage anatomy—all of our ribcage is not made of bone. (Figure 6-A) The front third, both left and right of our breastbone (sternum), is cartilage—a stout, sturdy material that is not infiltrated with calcium and **doesn't visualize** on x-rays. Athletes can quite commonly "pop" the costochondral junction where the bony rib and the cartilage struts are spot-welded together. This is a weak point in the circular ribcage.

MECHANISM OF INJURY

Wrestlers and grapplers are exposed to unique situations that create a high incidence of costochondral tears. Few sports create the mechanism of injury wherein violent TORSIONAL STRESSES are gen-

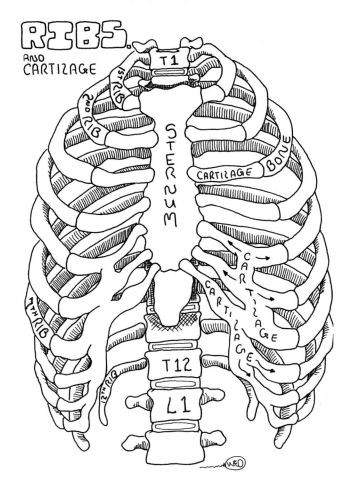

Figure 6-A: Ribcage anatomy

erated while a constrained athlete twists his pinned body to escape a hold. He can "pop" the costochondral junction. Additionally, the wrestler is subject to THE DIRECT COMPRESSION FORCES of his opponent's body weight as one falls upon the other's ribcage. I reported these mechanisms in 1980 in *The Physician and SportsMedicine* within a scientific article entitled "Injuries in Interscholastic Wrestling." My review of 666 wrestling injuries analyzed the mechanisms of injury, levels of recovery, and durations of disability. Chest injuries composed 5% of all wrestling injuries. (Out of interest the usual location of wrestling injuries is listed below).

KNEE	38.4%
SHOULDER	16.2%
EAR	7.6%
MISC.	7.1%
BACK	6.2%
HEAD & NECK	5.7%
ELBOW	5.0%
HAND	5.0%
CHEST	5.0%
ANKLE	3.9%

My career has also allowed me to report on the injuries sustained by 81 wrestlers in the 1976 United States Olympic Trials. 14% of these reported wrestling injuries occurred to the chest. Seven participants sustained costo-chondral sprains while one fractured a rib.

It is quite obvious that a DIRECT PUNCH, elbow, or kick to the ribs can crack a rib. This x-ray (Figure 6-B) demonstrates an actual fracture that occurred during the USA Boxing National Championships. A boxer may bravely and halfheartedly continue a bout until another solid follow-up punch lands. So much consuming effort is expended keeping elbows tucked in to protect that he becomes a sitting duck. One can't generate torque to return a solid punch with traumatized ribs. The bottom line is—a cracked rib immediately ends an encounter or very shortly leads to defeat. My physical exam for boxing includes side-to-side and front-to-back pressure on the athlete's ribcage. Even tough guys will wince and grimace if attempting to fool me by hiding an injury.

If I suspect a rib injury, an x-ray is routinely ordered. A confirmed fracture allows me to accurately predict a 6 to 8

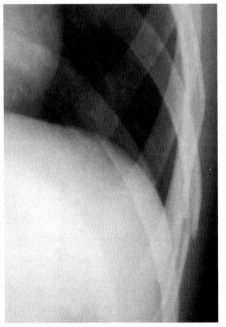

Figure 6-B: X-ray of fractured rib

week recovery period. If a rib is bruised and not demonstrated as broken on x-ray, a shorter recovery is probable. Here is where a knowledge of anatomy comes in handy. If the x-ray is negative but all of the pain is located along the nipple line (costochondral junctions), a 6 to 8 week recovery time also results. X-ray evaluation also allows the doctor to rule out associated lung injury such as a punctured lung or fluid within the chest. Your doctor can also count the number of involved ribs.

The mechanisms of injury to the ribcage thus include:

1. A direct blow—A punch, kick
2. Compression—A weighted fall onto the ribs
3. Torque—A sharp twist to change body alignment

TREATMENT

If you have a sharp pin-point soreness that interferes with your breathing, seek advice from a sportsmedicine doc. Should you actually feel a grating, clicking, rubbing, or popping of the ribs as you move or breathe, expect that a rib has (ribs have) been broken.

Refresher time: REMEMBER THAT BROKEN, FRACTURED, AND CRACKED HAVE IDENTICAL MEANINGS. THEY ARE SYNONYMS.

The routine, basic methods of care include:

1. Obtain an x-ray evaluation as explained before.

2. Pain medications. I advise that my patients—however tough and stoic—utilize some form of analgesic for the initial one or two weeks. If injury causes one to breathe shallowly and the lungs are not normally inflated, fluid and secretions can collect causing pneumonia. Occasional deep breathing and light coughing are normal, every-day functions that keep our lungs clean and healthy. Failure to expand the ribcage and cleanse the pipes creates infection—pneumonia. A secondary case of pneumonia will hamper your comeback much more extensively than just cracked ribs. Your goal consists of the ability to aerate your lungs to a reasonably normal degree. Too large a dose of narcotic will sedate and additionally interfere with normal healthy breathing. Moderation rules again.

3. Rib belts are very useful! Some doctors disagree with their benefits. I constantly and consistently return to my highly reliable form of research

and scientific investigation: ASK THE PATIENT! Many patients have confirmingly thanked me for supplying them with this form of splint after coming to my office empty-handed (bare-chested) from the emergency room. It does help me to seek the patient's opinion. All docs aren't pompous, close-minded, egotistical fools. The instructions for proper fit are simple (Figure 6-C)—too loose and it won't help—too tight and you can't breathe.

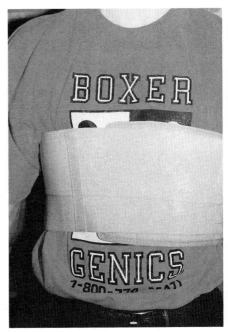

Figure 6-C: Rib belt

4. **Use temperance in your physical activity levels** for about 6 to 8 weeks. Light exercise and walking will be tolerated in several weeks. Twisting and turning which generate torque on the ribs should be avoided until full healing occurs.

5. Ice applied locally to the injured ribs will contribute pain relief in the initial few days.

6. All of this recovery information applies to both cracked ribs and sprained costochondral cartilage junctions.

7. The sudden onset of difficult breathing and shortness of breath **(assuming no heart conditions),** can suggest a popped lung (pneumothorax). In this emergency situation, air has escaped from inside the traumatized lung and is now "free air" causing the lung to collapse—"your balloon has popped." Emergency treatment is required to reinflate the lung and remove the negative pressure from inside the chest wall. (Figure 6-D)

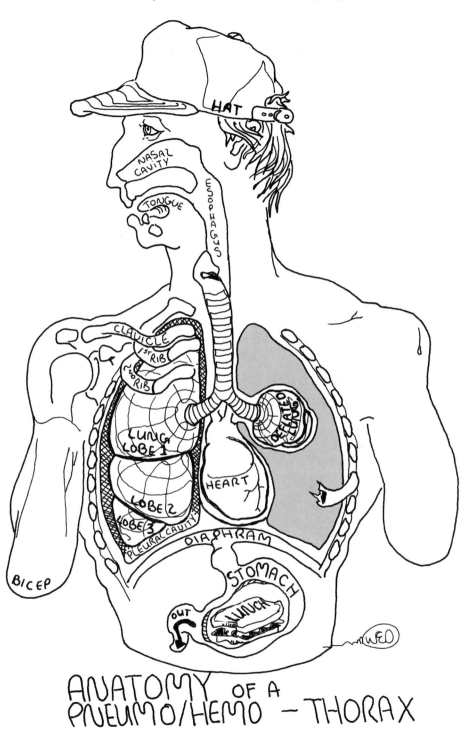

Figure 6-D: Collapsed lung — "Your balloon has popped!"

BREAST INJURY

Controversy and folklore abound when the topics of female boxing, full contact fighting, and proper protective gear surface.

What injuries will women suffer?

What happens if the breast tissue is traumatized?

Will it lead to cancer?

How much protection is needed?

A brief historical review may uncomplicate my answers. In 1993, a talented 16 year old female pianist successfully sued United States Amateur Boxing to become the first female to compete in an officially sanctioned bout. A female judge in Oregon placed USA Boxing under court order and penalty until the bout commenced. This ground-breaking young lady competed once, then retired. A group from USA Boxing's Sportsmedicine Committee, of which I was chairman, hustled to create rules and overnight guidelines for safe participation. We literally sat around a table in a hotel lobby drawing upon our combined past experiences as the competition guidelines were formulated by emergency legislation. Once the crisis was handled, we academically regrouped to gather professional opinion from national experts on women in sport. The extremely volatile concern that women would now be exposed to abdominal punches created questions about fertility and pregnancy. Were ovaries and womb sheltered from bombardment?

On the issue of breast trauma, an understanding of basic biologic principles diffuses confusing hype and hysteria. Let's separate fact from fiction! REPEATED TRAUMA TO THE BREAST WILL NOT CAUSE CANCER. Why? No co-existing scientific tissue model exists to support this folklore. Do blows to the abdominal muscles of men cause stomach muscle cancer? Do repeated punches on a heavy bag cause cancers to pop out all over the knuckles of the karate experts? Even if they break boards? No. No. No. Blunt trauma to tissues has not been recognized to influence a cancerous transformation. A complication might potentially arise since a tender hematoma could confuse the examiner of a breast mass. However, the history of competition and the rapid resolution of the firm area should simplify diagnosis.

It is entirely appropriate and judicious that some form of female chest padding is recommended. I suggest that no hard plastic compounds are used so that punchers don't suffer hand or finger injury. I additionally suggest that the protective shield be limited to cover only the breast area and not excessively cover the entire abdominal area. If valid stomach punches are prevented, the opponent might be encouraged to become a "head hunter." An excessive proportion of blows will then be aimed at the lesser protected head region. Keep our priorities straight. Don't sacrifice the brain for unfounded, over-protective concerns about the trunk.

Gynecological experts assure us that a woman's ovaries and even a first trimester pregnant uterus are effectively protected within the bony ring of the pelvis. One national expert graphically punctuated her point by sarcastically noting that the male of the species is at greatest "glandular risk" during combat. If reproductive concerns are valid, the men "hang out" at far greater consequence. Despite her anatomical wisdom, fight promoters must wisely disqualify any female competitor who, however remote, could be pregnant. The safety of an innocent third person is not to be remotely endangered during sports competition.

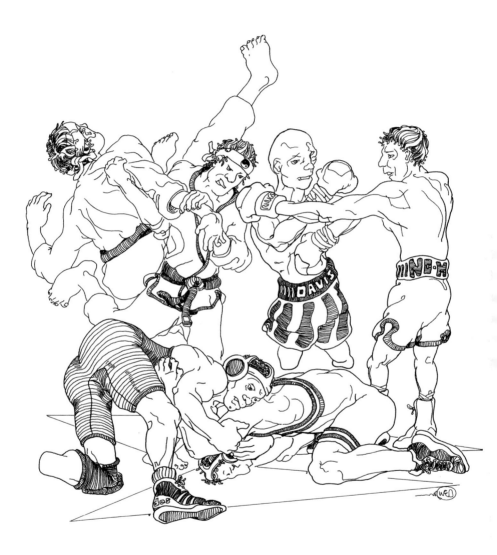

Chapter 7

Abdominal Injuries
In the Combat Arts

Abdominal injuries may uncommonly occur in the combat arts. Although any organ in the abdomen may be injured, the signs and symptoms of these injuries are often similar. Many of these symptoms can be very subtle yet reflect serious injury. A qualified physician, therefore, should examine individuals with potential abdominal organ injury. The most common symptoms that may occur in these injuries are abdominal pain, nausea, vomiting (with or without blood), and splinting of the abdomen due to pain. Various organs in the abdomen may be susceptible to injury.

KIDNEYS

The kidneys are somewhat superficial targets damaged by blows to the upper abdomen and/or flank areas. A tear in the kidney may lead to life threatening internal bleeding. A kidney injury should always be suspected if one alertly notices bloody or dark colored urine. These individuals should be checked by a physician who may order special ultrasound scans, dye studies, or computer x-rays to determine if an operation is necessary to repair the damage. A possible late complication of kidney injury includes high blood pressure, so at-risk individuals should be watched closely for this problem.

SPLEEN AND LIVER

The spleen and liver are susceptible to the blunt-trauma punches, kicks, and falls that may occur during the combat sports. A competitor already subjected to the complications of infectious mononucleosis is more likely to sustain internal organ damage. In people with "mono," the spleen is enlarged. This swollen spleen may be ruptured by either a direct blow or by straining during strenuous activities. With a ruptured spleen, the athlete experiences a sudden onset of pain and tenderness mainly in the left upper abdomen. Pain may also radiate into the left shoulder and be worsened by deep breathing. As a consequence of massive bleeding, the exerciser may be pale, light headed, and then collapse. Persons with a ruptured spleen should obviously be ambulanced to a health care facility as an emergency.

Due to this possible complication, it is recommended that those with mono should delay participating in light, non-strenuous exercise until at least three weeks after their illness, assuming that their spleen has not markedly enlarged per physician examination. For strenuous and contact sports, these lesser involved cases may resume activity approximately one month after their illness. If an athlete's spleen is found to be enlarged by palpation during examination, a significant rest period must be safely fulfilled until cleared by medical advice.

The liver may be damaged by a blow to the upper right abdomen. (Figure 7-A and Figure 7-B) A fractured lower right rib may cause a tear in the liver. A lacerated or damaged liver will cause symptoms similar to a ruptured spleen, but on the right side instead of the left. These injuries should also be seen immediately by a physician.

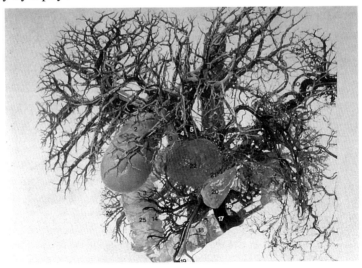

Figure 7-A: Vascularity of the liver

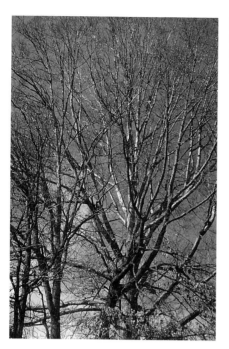

Figure 7-B: Photo of tree (to compare to liver). Doesn't the architecture of nature work in beautifully similar patterns?

Any abdominal injury may cause the athlete to develop an "acute abdomen" with severe pain. These situations present quite a challenge at ringside and the better part of valor simply requires the **suspicion** of serious injury, not an **exact** confirmatory diagnosis. Recognize a problem and ship it out! The patient should be stabilized and transported to the nearest emergency room. Repeat examinations are necessary when suspicion of an internal injury exists.

SPECIAL SITUATIONS

Though injuries to the pancreas, mesentery, omentum, and bladder are possible, they are not common. Because such injuries may be difficult to diagnose, a delay in recognition and treatment can occur, and therefore proper medical observation is mandatory. Let us discuss a few situations:

PANCREAS

The pancreas was commonly injured in the horse and buggy era by horses that kicked their grooms in the upper abdomen. Blows from the foot or hand to a relaxed abdominal wall may cause such an injury to the pancreas, though highly unlikely in boxing or the martial arts.

MESENTERY AND OMENTUM

The mesentery is the scaffold that supports blood vessels to the gut and it can be injured with resultant hematoma. Harm does not always result. The omentum is the "policeman" of the abdomen because it protects injured areas, especially if infection is the cause. The omentum itself may be injured. These contusions and hematomas are usually not serious.

BLADDER

It would be rare for the bladder to be injured in either boxing or the martial arts. However, a bladder filled with urine can be contused with subsequent bleeding. Rupture is more serious and may cause an acutely distended abdomen to develop. This is highly unlikely. Always empty your bladder prior to actual competitive participation or rigorous training.

Injuries to the bladder, genitals, and testicles are unlikely especially if a protective cup is worn.

LOW BLOWS

Unfortunately, punches and kicks that land in the groin area prematurely end, or controversially influence, the outcome of otherwise competitive bouts. Fortunately, self-defense strikes to this vulnerable target zone by an undersized victim can salvage a treacherous, vicious attack situation.

In order to understand this gut-wrenching, breath-holding, eye-bulging effect, you need to understand early human anatomy and development. Within the young male embryo, the testicles actually develop within the abdominal cavity near the kidneys and intestines. In those final months before birth, the infant's testicles gradually descend out of his abdomen and into the scrotal sac. Despite their journey, the two testicles retain and share some of the same nerves that innervate a variety of abdominal structures. This is the basis for the nausea and deep sickening internal pains that prominently accompany "low" blows. A vaso-vagal nerve response (sweating, dizziness, fainting, low blood pressure) can also complicate the internal pain or visceral response.

What's the best and worst scenario? Most responses are intense but brief and rarely cause short-term or long-term consequences. The testes and scrotum are so mobile that they usually escape true crushing, direct injury. Mor dangerous, is an upward kick that catches the tissues between a broad foot and the bones of the pelvis. Other more serious complications include hematomas, secondary inflammation of the tubes surrounding the testicles, and testicular rupture. Rupture or tearing of the actual testicle is a serious event requiring medical specialist attention.

What can we do to help? I have witnessed all sorts of witchcraft, folklore, and "I've got to do something" reactions. One of the most amusing occurred last year as I sat at ringside witnessing a minor low blow that landed seconds before the end of an early round. The impact was minimal. The recipient remained standing and defensively maintained his position making it to his corner as the bell rang, signaling his one-minute, between round, rest period. I was not concerned for his safety. The blow was real but glanced off in a minor manner. What I'll describe next is the original "water bottle" cure. Traditionally, the corner man and coach cool the weary, sweaty competitor by toweling him off, tending to cuts, rinsing his mouthpiece, giving a small swallow of water, and pouring a portion of the water bottle over his head to cool him down. All of this occurs during a fleeting one-minute flurry of instructions, scolding, or psych-up. The mildly grimacing boxer still experiencing some level of discomfort looked to his coaches for last second miracles. Doing "what comes naturally" and in a "we've got to do something" mode, they gently tugged on his no-foul groin protector and proceeded to empty the remainder of the water bottle down his trunks. Not surprisingly, he straightened his legs, jerked his head up and nearly landed in the center of the ring. I don't know if he was in fighting shape but he somehow felt safer in the ring than in his corner. I guess they reasoned that if water works on the head, it might work down below!

What should we really do in such a situation? My consultation and advice from urologists suggests the following:

1. Allow the competitor to remain lying down if he has already dropped down. A vaso-vagal response stimulated by the pain can lower one's blood pressure causing fainting. Treat this initial phase with the same principles as if treating mild shock or fainting.

2. You will notice that a stricken athlete will tend to draw-up into the fetal position. One instinctively does this to relax the stomach muscles and

take the stretch off the abdominal contents. Remember your anatomy lesson! Allow the athlete lying on his back to bend his knees and further relax the muscles.

3. Encourage slow, deep breathing.

4. Gently loosen the padded groin protector to ease pressure.

Don't panic for miracle cures at ringside. There are no quick fixes. The speed of recovery is related to the force of the blow.

After his exit from the ring, mat, or arena, I suggest:

1. He continue wearing a properly fitted jock strap or athletic supporter.

2. Apply a well insulated ice pack if a hematoma is developing.

3. Use Tylenol or anti-inflammatories if appropriate for pain.

4. If significant symptoms last for greater than one hour, consult a physician. You may be referred to a urologist who specializes in this aspect of medicine.

CELIAC PLEXUS

This dense network of anatomic nerves is located in the upper abdomen near the spine. Its branches are distributed to the organs mentioned earlier and controls vasomotor tone to these organs. Injuries to the plexus can cause fainting, weakness, and temporary collapse thus mandating the usual emergency vigilance to assist the athlete.

GROIN PULLS

Strained groin muscles commonly occur in all sports, especially combat arts that include kicking. Problems occur when the muscles on the inner thigh are stretched too far, too fast. Activity or movements that cause this injury include slipping while the legs are being forced apart or when over-extending a kick. The individual experiences sudden pain, a cramp-like ache as the torn muscle segments contract and spasm, and possible swelling on the inner thigh. Several days later a bruise may appear on the skin several inches away from the actual and deeper muscle injury. The bleeding from the torn muscle fibers surfaces on the skin after gravity carries the bruise several inches from the site of tear.

Treatment for this injury includes rest, ice, and compression. This is followed by rehabilitation with strength and flexibility exercises to protect from further injury. Activity can often be resumed earlier if the thigh is wrapped with an elastic bandage or a specially designed Neoprene or elastic thigh sleeve is worn. Groin pulls can be confused with hip problems, pelvic stress fractures, hernias, and pubic symphysis injury.

CARING FOR SUSPECTED ABDOMINAL INJURIES

1. Referees must remain vigilant and protect the athlete at all times.

2. Consult the ringside doctor often during a bout if trouble is suspected.

3. Determine levels of alertness at ringside.

4. Conduct a rapid ringside examination, and then retreat to a locker room where a more private, unhurried exam can be continued.

5. Remember that the status of the airway, breathing, and cardiac systems takes priority.

6. Administer oxygen when appropriate. Be certain oxygen is supplied for full contact fights/bouts. Always **check the pressure** of the facility's oxygen tank before the competitions begin. Don't trust the word of promoters, etc. I have personally discovered the tanks of major city arenas to be out of date and totally out of pressure!

7. Watch for inappropriate breathing patterns. Normal breathing - chest out, abdomen out. Abnormal breathing - chest out, abdomen not out. Suspect abdominal injury.

8. Check urine sample, if possible, for bleeding. Send this information to the hospital.

9. If in doubt about an athlete's status, transport to the nearest emergency facility and confirm that he is seen by a qualified general surgeon.

10. The responsible coach, trainer, doctor, and family should follow the progress of the injured athlete in the hospital setting and learn from the experience precipitating the injury.

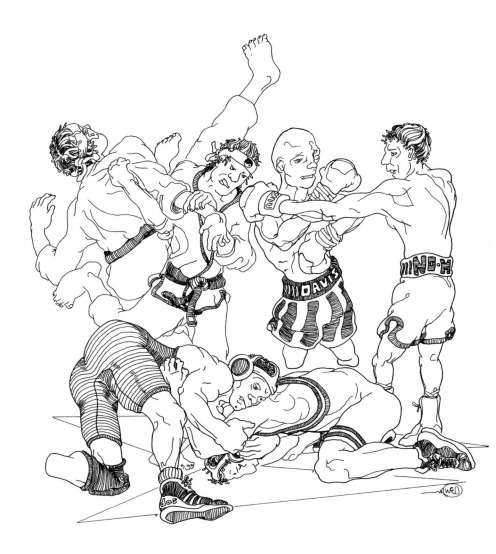

Chapter 8

Head and Neck Injury

CONCUSSION AND HOW TO MONITOR SYMPTOMS

It happened to me just last week! Actually, I should say that it happened to him—our boxer. While overseas in London for an international bout, one of our boxers was knocked out. As an accompanying ringside physician, shoulder the responsibility of our team's safety. The opportunity to travel nternationally with a team is great fun until the big-fisted clock strikes the our and the bouts begin. Suddenly it's show time and anxiety, alertness, and esponsibility take precedence over the travel distractions. When one occu-ies the "hot-seat," desires for ferocious battles conservatively wilt into hopes or a boring evening. I don't want injuries!

Alex was a young boxer and not experienced enough to confront a former ational champion of England. Our elite coach barely had enough time to ana-yze the developing bout as Alex was leveled early in the first round—too early or our coach to decisively quit and throw in the towel. A solid right hand elivered the "lights out" blow. It landed quickly and with authority. Our boxer idn't see it coming. Backward he toppled, as if falling off a log. Dangerous-y, he fell between the bottom and next-to-bottom ropes. His head and neck ere whipped further backward towards the crowd as the bottom rope vibrat-d in response to his body weight. Alex rolled off the ropes by the angulation f his own body weight. As I scurried up the steps, through the ropes, and cross to the opposite side of the ring, he lay on his back and was unmoving. lis predicament became potentially two-fold, blatantly delineating what companion injuries must be anticipated in every unconscious fighter. ASSUME THAT A NECK INJURY IS ALSO PRESENT IN EVERY UNCONSCIOUS COMBAT PARTICIPANT.

Many a boxer is rendered "out on his feet," "lights out," standing. Being knocked-out is bad enough, but gravity has yet to exert its powerful follow-up punch. Any head injury is compounded by the additional forces generated by the mat, ropes, and awkward falls. For this very reason, tournament personnel should demand modern materials, proper maintenance, and secure assembly of competition sites!

What to do now? Hardly a mystery! This scenario has been practiced, rehearsed, and performed on many occasions during my career as a ringside physician. I have supervised greater than 10,000 bouts. Let me share with you the things I look for and am always concerned about.

The big picture for safety priority is as follows:

ESSENTIAL FIRST AID FOR COMBAT INJURY—A, B, C, D'S

Airway—Is he mechanically positioned to allow for the unobstructed inflow-outflow of air?

Breathing—Is he breathing on his own?

Circulation—Is his heart pumping effectively?

Disability—What is his level of consciousness? Is he oriented and can he move all limbs? How long is he out?

Skeletal—Are his head, neck, spinal cord, or extremities injured? Can he be moved in any manner? Must he be moved?

My mind has been trained to orderly race through these critical criteria for severity of injury. As a fellow athlete, coach, trainer, or referee, you will be required to make judgments also. Docs aren't always around for training room injuries. Let's hope you request medical supervision of boxing matches and martial arts tournaments. Wrestling tournaments can certainly accumulate their share of trauma.

I was concerned about Alex's neck because he bounced about on the lower ringside rope. Only when the athlete moves all extremities and wakes up to confirm the absence of neck pain can you allow unprotected neck movement

routinely palpate along the athlete's neck to search for sore vertebrae. If the athlete remains unconscious and in an awkward posture, a **team effort** is used to log roll the patient into a straightened position. The **most experienced person controls the head and neck** so that all movements are conducted with coordinated rotation alignment to the body. Longitudinal straight, gentle, direct traction on the neck is maintained. Minimize your movements. Once maneuvered into an accessible alignment, the other critical considerations are addressed. Thankfully his vacant stare evolved into eye blinking, a limp body began slowly bending knees and elbows, and this silent youth started asking "Where am I?" The recovering emergence from cocoon to fluttering butterfly can transform in slow seconds. My anxiety drops equally fast. In my performance of duty, I'm sure that I was less aware of the onlooking crowd than our knocked-out boxer. It's always like that if you concentrate on your job. The pre-game jitters fade as the competition actually commences and one must perform their trained activity.

The natural tendency of a knocked-out athlete is to salvage his pride and jump up to prove his invincibility. Not so fast! A step-wise mobilization uncovers lesser injuries that readily become apparent—a dislocated shoulder, injured ribs, twisted knee, broken jaw. First, allow the fallen warrior to sit up on the canvas. Progress him to sitting on a stool. Return him to the coaches in his corner. Don't make a big deal out of the process. Proceed along and assist him out of the ring for a detailed, unrushed, unpressured exam. Alex quickly regained orientation and balance. He confirmed that he never saw the punch develop or arrive. His duration of unconsciousness lasted about 20 seconds by my estimation, realizing that one usually overestimates in these situations, seconds seem like minutes. Have the timekeeper actually use a stopwatch to record the time period of unconsciousness. He extended a conciliatory handshake to his opponent and exited the ring on his own power. His risks and my exams were not over. He deserved follow-up surveillance that evening and the next day by doc, coaches, and roommates.

Thank God that serious injury rarely occurs in competitions. My most hair-raising situation occurred thanks to Kertis. When I do occasionally meet Kertis, I remind him that he assumes full responsibility for my first gray hair. He had one hell of a punch! Once, in the dark, dingy V. F. W. hall of a 5,000-person town, Kertis punched a guy so hard, he was unconscious standing-up. As soon as he toppled like a chain-sawed tree and bounced like a deflating ball— the seizures started. I'm talking grand mal, eyes rolled up, no breathing, turning blue, uncontrolled limb flailing type. It can happen! Two of us docs were in attendance, had oxygen available, and protected him through the 45-second ordeal. He was ushered by ambulance to the hospital, brain scanned, admitted for overnight observation, and discharged for follow-up by a neurologist. We unarguably banned him for any future competitions. I will never cover a boxing or full contact martial arts event without ambulance, oxygen and transport personnel in attendance. Phone communication must be available. I advise that any ringside doctor do the same. No amount of knowledge and experience can compensate for modern equipment and comprehensive facilities. A well trained doctor is stranded on a deserted island without his sophisticated tools. Parents should serve as watchdogs for their children's safety. Promoters must assume comprehensive responsibility for contingency plans—give free tickets, hot dogs, soft drinks, and hats to neighboring volunteer firefighters or ambulance squads. Make them feel welcome and a vital part of the team and event.

MECHANISM OF HEAD INJURY

First, I'll explain what happened when—"The lights went out. " The brain floats in a rock solid vault called the skull. I often, however, use the analogy of a yolk (brain) suspended in its shell (skull). One doesn't have to crack a skull in order to suffer brain injury. Shaking an egg violently can scramble the yolk without cracking its shell. On the other hand, a sharp tap on the edge of the frying pan can totally open a shell without breaking the yolk. Accomplished cooks can successfully duplicate this feat with their eyes closed. Punches, kicks, head butts, or elbows delivered by an opponent to the head produce a sudden acceleration which shakes and scrambles the yolk within its intact shell. This scrambling interferes with the transmission of nerve impulses, short circuiting the brain cells, leading to an altered state of consciousness. Certain blows create a more rapid acceleration of the head than others. The classic angular or rotational accelerated knock-out punch is delivered by either an upper cut or a cross. (Figure 8-A) These alter the brain functions with more intensity than straight punches. Obviously, any powerfully

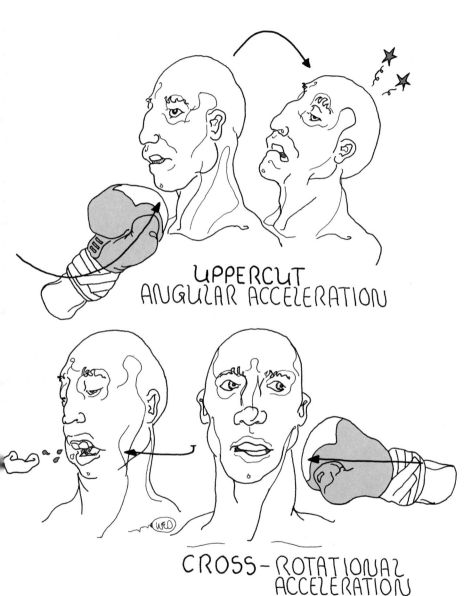

Figure 8-A: Upper cut and cross punches

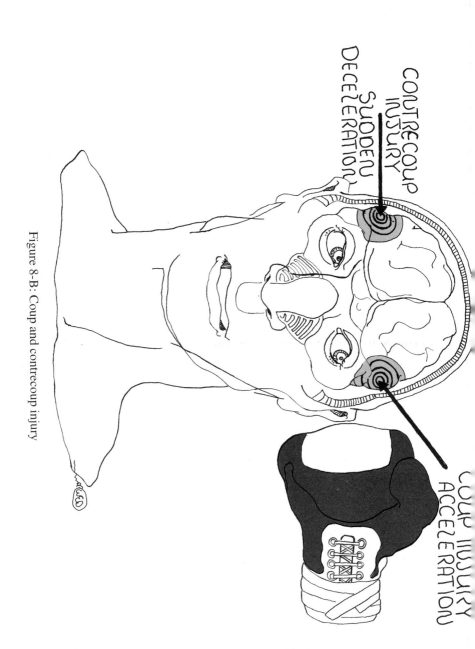

Figure 8-B: Coup and contrecoup injury

absorbed head punch or kick carries the potential to knock-out, maim, or destroy an opponent.

The initial effect of a knock-out punch "temporarily" halts brain message transmissions. More about "temporary" later! Any additional impact forces may actually bruise a surface of our jello-like brain. Quite often the sloshing motion of the **accelerated** brain actually results in a bruise to the opposite side of the brain as it bounces back against the skull in a **deceleration** mode. Rapid acceleration and deceleration movements each create havoc, resulting in what we call **coup** (direct) and **contrecoup** (indirect/opposite) injury. (Figure 8-B) A properly padded ring mat and headgear can limit the secondary contrecoup and deceleration forces as a boxer drops to the floor. Research has not claimed that headgear can abolish the acceleration forces that precipitate brain injury. It is, however, reasonable to expect that additional forces from an unconscious fall to the mat may be dissipated. An early study of amateur boxers by Dr. Mickey Demos reported 22% of head injuries occurring in boxers while wearing headgear and 78% of head injuries occurring in those not utilizing headgear. In defense of headgear usage, facial cuts have been dramatically reduced by the legislated wearing of headgear by amateur boxers. During the five day 1996 Olympic Boxing Trials, we did not need to treat or suture a single laceration thanks to the use of headgear.

Even with the distinct viewing advantage of sitting directly at ringside during a bout, it is nearly impossible to make judgments based on a fighter's pupils. The only individual with a close-up view is the referee. He must be well qualified and con-

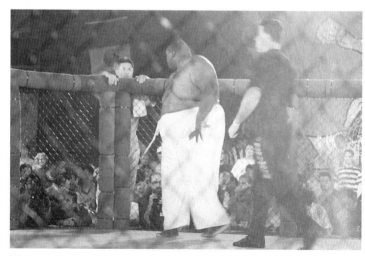

Figure 8-C: "Big" John McCarthy of Ultimate Fighting Championships (UFC)

scientious. In boxing, the officials keep score, and the primary responsibilities of the referee are: (1) the **safety** of the competitor, and (2) enforcing the **rules** of the sport.

I have been very impressed by the very competent refs, "Big" John McCarthy of the Ultimate Fighting Championships (Figure 8-C), active competitor John Donehue of Extreme Fighting, and the legendary Cecil Peoples of The World Combat Championships who maintain deep concern for their combatants despite the advertised "no holds barred" aura. Only refs can maintain an intimate view and an instantaneous response to events.

Bart Vale, a world champion shoot fighter, recently withdrew from The World Combat Championship Tournament due to injuries. Afterwards he discussed with reporters his respect for my recommendation that he withdraw from the tournament. During our pre-event team meeting, the directors of The World Combat Championships supportively pronounced to the fighters that "in the ring the ref is God, outside the ring the doctor is God. " Bout organizers can legislate that safety remains supreme, and that decisions made in the spirit of safety will be fully supported. Full contact and Reality events do ultimately have rules, however unspoken or unadvertised. A mutual respect and rapport allowed both John's, Cecil, and me to maintain eye contact and instantaneous communication despite that intimidating, chain-link fenced, circle of combat. We had our game plan.

Outside the confines of any ring, there remain solidly effective methods for monitoring a performer's level of alertness. I can't see his eyes, but I can watch his feet. A highly tuned machine that runs out of gas will cease precision movements, sputter, and stumble. A wide-based stance for compensated stability predicts trouble. Loss of crispness, slow ring movement, flat-footedness fatigue, and leaning on the opponent (clinching) suggest problems. You can tell a lot about a boxer's head by observing his feet.

I can't see the eyes, but I can watch his/her hands. (Figure 8-D) Uncharacteristic lowering of the hands suggests loss of trained basics. Loss of crisp punches is as predictive as a warning bell. The overpoweringly blatant reason to halt a bout arrives when an athlete is **no longer able to adequately protect herself/himself.** (Figure 8-E) The contest is no longer a contest when this occurs. *(See Chapter Two for more detailed hints).*

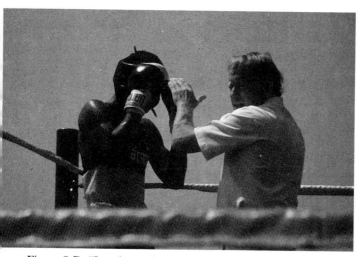

Figure 8-D: "I can't see the eyes, but I can watch his hands"

The standing 8-count, when allowed, constitutes a very useful tool to monitor safety. The 8-count does not belong to the athlete. This was not meant as a time-out for him to catch his breath or wits. This is a referee's tool to allow a more uninterrupted, intense observation of the athlete.

When rules and circumstances allow, I value the opportunity to ascend up to the ring or mat and personally examine the competitor. Solid medical decisions can result from this short, but pertinent review. Many times an athlete is found to be clear-headed and focused which confirms the ability to continue. On other occasions, I have found a broken hand, broken nose, or eyes that cross, and two minds that don't meet on this same planet. One of my most humbling experiences in boxing occurred as I was requested by the ref to examine an injured boxer during USA Boxing's National Championship Tournament. Scampering up the wobbly steps, I was simultaneously putting on exam gloves, balancing flashlight, and opening gauze sponges. I was just four months post knee surgery myself. I slipped and fell while bounding up those steps. My tools were gathered and I limpingly continued up to the bleeding boxer and senior referee who patiently witnessed my near T. K. O. With my wounded ego, I was stunned and surprised when former Olympic official (and friend) Marco Sarfaraz turned his attention from the bloody-nosed boxer and directed a ceremoniously formal eight-count to **me** in front of the appreciative arena. We all had a laugh. I cleared the boxer and limped down the stairs to tend to my pride and bleeding shin.

RINGSIDE OBSERVATION
(MONITORING SAFETY)

"I can't see his eyes, but I can watch his <u>feet</u>"! (1996)

    1.   Stance - skill level, balance

    2.   Ring movement - dominance or "running"

"I can't see her eyes, but I can watch her <u>hands</u>"! (1996)

    3.   Defense - "ultimate determinate", (1979 McCown) - "A one-sided contest should be halted minutes early, rather than seconds late".

    4.   Punch Count - flow of bout

    5.   Lowered Arms - fatigue, body blows

<u>Fatigue</u> Factors

    6.   Clinches

    7.   Number of 8 counts

    8.   "Bruise" news - accumulating trauma

<u>Extraneous</u> Factors

    9.   Referee's Level of Attentiveness

    10.   Corner Activity - rest periods and during bout

Figure 8-E: Chart of Ringside Observation (monitoring safety)

CHRONIC BRAIN INJURY

What really happens as the multiple folds of brain slosh back and forth like waves crashing on a rocky coast? Can it sink our ship? Yes! Traumatized cells can die in numbers that capsize our ship. Certain areas of the brain seem particularly sensitive to multiple insults. Minor concussions sustained over a great period of time, create a recognized **cumulative** effect labeled DEMENTIA PUGILISTICA—"punch drunk." It is a very real entity that surfaces deceivingly slowly later in life after repeated insults. This may be thought of as post-injury "arthritis of the brain"! We often do not realize the pounding our knees and backs have accumulated until years after football and soccer careers have ended. These brain injuries are felt to be cumulative, like x-ray or sun exposure, so that each "bell rung" may never be entirely forgotten or forgiven.

Pathologists have dissected the brains of boxers confirmed to have suffered dementia. The gross and microscopic evidence has actually confirmed the following brain alterations:

1. CEREBRAL ATROPHY & DILATATION OF VENTRICLES—this may result in senility and loss of intellect.

2. CEREBELLUM CHANGES—this may cause poor balance.

3. PERFORATED SEPTUM PELLUCIDUM (CEREBRUM)—this may lead to impaired memory and emotional instability.

4. DEGENERATION OF SUBSTANTIA NIGRA—this may contribute to Parkinson's syndrome.

The rather direct correlation of behavior characteristics and related cell scaring in boxers leaves little doubt about cause and effect. Protect yourself from repeated blows to the head. Learn and practice defensive techniques. Compete at a level consistent with your skills. Train under a trusted coach who level-headedly looks out for your best long-term interest. He must know when to throw-in the towel because a competitor rarely quits in the ring or on the mat. Dr. Barry Jordan has summarized the risk factors for dementia pugilistica in the many pro boxers he has evaluated for the New York State Athletic Commission as:

1. Duration of career
2. Age at retirement
3. Win - loss record
4. Total number of bouts
5. Age at time of examination

I know a 40 year old former pro boxer who brags that he has fought the best and been K. O. 'd by two world champions. One may be initially impressed until being personally subjected to his brain-dead babble. Slurred speech, unsteady gait, and boringly repeated words and sentences don't promote a pleasant conversation. I avoid getting cornered into meaningless jabber with him. Sadly, he slides from job to job while responsible for a devoted wife and straight-A-student son. Incidentally, his gifted son is nationally ranked as an amateur boxer within his age group. Let's hope he doesn't absorb the punishment that his father glorifies.

More input on exposure risks. Your chance of developing skin cancer closely relates to your body's total accumulated dose of sun exposure as a child and teenager. Numerous severe sunburns and skin peelings significantly impact your statistics. Cells begin aging from the moment we are born. Unfortunate exposures cause premature aging. Use sensible precautions when competing as a fighter. Learn good offensive and defensive techniques. Sun blocking agents shield our skin, punch blocking shields our brain.

Researchers in Virginia have performed a prospective study of mild head injury in college football players. The technique of **neuropsychological** testing has proven the most accurate for documenting brain dysfunction following concussion—better than EEG, CAT scans, MRI scans, or PET scans.

Neuropsychologic—Memory testing and analysis of brain skills such as mathematics and calculations

EEG—Electroencephalogram (electric brain waves)

CAT scan—Computerized axial tomography (x-rays that are computerized for greater detail)

MRI scan—Magnetic resonance imaging (the use of magnetic fields instead of x-ray exposure for computerized images)

PET scan—Positron emission tomography (a powerful isotope investigation technique for the study of the physiology, pathology, and pharmacology of the brain)

Evaluation of 195 injuries, *Mild Head Injury* by Harvey S. Levin, Ph. D. , suggested that "single mild head injury in football players often causes cognitive/information processing deficits which can be documented on neuropsychological assessment within 24 hours of the insult, and that rapid, although perhaps incomplete, recovery may take place over the next 5 to 10 days." It seems appropriate to apply these college studies to amateur athletes in the combat sports. We know that the trend suggests prolonged trouble after multiple insults, i. e. , "dementia athletica," but we don't have long term specifics for the amateur athlete. The Johns Hopkins study did comfort those in amateur boxing.

The prestigious Johns Hopkins University coordinated a pre-eminent prospective study on amateur boxing. Data on 500 athletes in six major U. S. cities was compiled. After five years of focusing on the sport of Olympic-style boxing, the following conclusions were reached:

1. No statistically significant changes in visuoconstructional abilities nor memory were found after baseline determinations.

2. Some pre-existing changes in memory function and visuoconstructional ability were found at baseline but there was no progression during the five year study. Questions remain as to why there was abnormality at the beginning of the study. Childhood injury? Educational level? Drugs? Cultural variation? Was the five year study too short to document changes?

3. The data collected thus far suggests that there is no link between participating in amateur/Olympic-style boxing and changes in central nervous system function.

4. Long term follow-up is recommended.

In essence, concussive brain injury is potentially additive and accumulative just as sunburn affects the aging of skin and the subsequent development of cancer. Parents and coaches cannot accept a casual approach to brain injury in their children just because "soccer is safe" and one wears a helmet during football. Having served as a team physician who stood on the sidelines for many football and soccer games, I am shocked at the multitude of uninformed misconceptions. My background in ringside physician responsibilities has provided a window to view contrasting parental sensitivity to head blows among sports. Head injury is correctly termed concussion in boxing, and sugar-coated in football as "bell ringing" or "dings." Don't think that subtle brain impact doesn't happen in soccer. "Heading" the ball includes the brain as an integral component of those redirecting forces. A rain-soaked soccer ball can weigh twice as much as a dry ball. When an amateur boxer sustains a significant head blow, USA Boxing rules require at least a 30-day suspension. The term, "the referee stops contest—head blow (RSC-H)," mandates a 30, 90, or 180 day non-competition period.

We have all heard the stories of the football player who:

1. Forgets the plays, runs the wrong direction

2. Is led back to his position by teammates

3. Is knocked out and returns for the second half

4. Suffers headaches after the game, then practices full contact on Monday.

Each of these circumstances signifies head (brain) injury. A boxer must rest 30 days. Let's hope that martial artists, soccer, and football players will equally respect the identical trauma to their brain cells. Listed here are the well developed guidelines established by USA Boxing. All contact sports should utilize these. (Figure 8-F)

Do not allow a return to competition or practice until all of these symptoms have resolved:

- Short term confusion
- Dizziness
- Unsteady gait
- Double vision
- Dazed
- Calculation ability: math, etc.
- Amnesia
- Memory ability: history, facts, etc.
- Headache
- Concentration
- Irritability

Our safest recommendation is to follow "Quigley's Rule" devised in 1973. Athletes should discontinue active participation in contact sports after receiving three cerebral concussions. Other researchers "contend that cognitive deficits are cumulative in successive concussions."

The "sleeper" in cumulative brain injury occurs during lesser scrutinized **practice sessions.** Greatest exposure to repeated injury occurs during training. Games, tournaments or bouts occupy a brief (although memorable) portion of an athlete's experience. The ringside or team doc is only present for a minuscule few minutes of an athlete's career. EACH COACH SHOULDERS A GOD-LIKE RESPONSIBILITY TO PROTECT HIS YOUTHFUL CHARGES. The teaching of technique is not his only responsibility. COACHES MUST FULLY UNDERSTAND THE APPLIED ANATOMY OF INJURY! A coach's perspective may become clouded by the regimentation of repetitious drills and exercises. They must get the big picture.

A lack of short-term recall about events **after** the injury is termed ANTEROGRADE MEMORY LOSS. For example, a fighter may actually win a bout but not know how he scored the winning blow. A football lineman may have successfully blocked-out the opposing tackle on a touchdown play yet not realize it until the game films are analyzed. The greater in duration the memory

---

RULES OF USA BOXING, INC.

RSCH
(REFEREE STOPS CONTEST - HEAD BLOW)

1. **RSCH-(30) - 30 day restriction period applies.** Examples are: three standing eight counts in one round or four in a bout due to head blows; a boxer who receives a stunning head blow and demonstrates a lack of normal response, but has not been knocked down; or a boxer who is knocked down from a head blow and immediately responds normally and assumes the upright, on-guard position, indicating intent to go on, however, the referee nevertheless stops the contest.

2. **RSCH-(90) - 90 day restriction period applies.** Examples are: a boxer who has been knocked unconscious and is unresponsive to normal stimuli for less than two minutes. The ringside physician shall determine the boxer's unresponsive time by consulting with the official timekeeper.

3. **RSCH-(180) - 180 day restriction period applies.** Examples are: a boxer who has been knocked unconscious and is unresponsive to normal stimuli for at least two minutes. The ringside physician shall determine the boxer's unresponsive time by consulting with the official timekeeper.

Figure 8-F: Rules of USA Boxing, Inc. regarding blows to the head

loss, the more severe the brain cell injury. In severe trauma, such as a knock-out, the duration of un- consciousness usually paral- lels the signifi- cance of brain injury. (Figure 8-G)

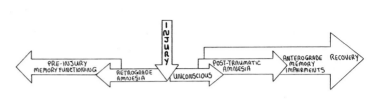

Figure 8-G: Retrograde and anterograde memory loss

Loss of memory for events **preceding** the injury is termed RETROGRADE memory loss. This deficit suggests significant injury. For example, the mar- tial artist who not only forgets what happened after the kick to his head, but also doesn't remember changing into his uniform before the tournament, defines great risk.

ACUTE BRAIN INJURY

The combat sports are risky but only in a relative sense. What are we com- paring them against? For a reality check, listed below are the number of deaths per 1,000 participants:

Horse Racing	128	Motorcycle Racing	7
Parachuting	126	High School/College Football	3
Hang Gliding	56	Boxing	1. 3
Scuba Diving	11		

What are the risks? So far, I have concentrated on explaining the long term concerns of accumulated brain injury that became so newsworthy in the great boxer Muhammed Ali. Let's remain quite aware that one can quickly die from that one single, significant blow to the head. Not only can we shake-up and scar brain cells, but we make them bleed. An extensive blood supply feeds and nourishes our "thinking cap. " Sudden blows can send that floating white and gray matter bouncing off the boney-hard walls of our skull. That violent shak- ing can tear abundant blood vessels.

Bleeding can happen rapidly or slowly. A rapid, arterial, high pressure blood clot is termed an EPIDURAL HEMATOMA. Death will rapidly occur. Remember, the skull doesn't have to be broken (fractured) for the brain to fatally bleed. The egg shell doesn't have to break for the yolk to be scrambled.

The more common serious accumulation of blood is termed a SUBDURAL HEMATOMA. Being venous and low pressure in origin, the growing clot develops its size more slowly—over hours or days instead of minutes. (Figure 8-H) The hard, unyielding skull and expanding clot finally and fatally squeeze the vital brain stem through a small hole at the bottom of our skull. You simulate this process daily as you squeeze viscous toothpaste from its protective tube and out through its small hole. A herniated lifeless brain assumes a similar consistency. The trick is recognizing and halting this pressure process before the fatal brain squeeze and shift. Rapid recognition of symptoms, transport to a hospital, x-ray documentation, and decompression surgery can prevent death and/or lingering sequelae. The pressure on the brain must be relieved before cells are permanently crushed. As the learned pioneer ringside physician Dr. McCown stated, "A one-sided contest should be halted minutes early, rather than seconds late. " Always error on the side of safety. Don't let a defenseless competitor risk injury. He/she may mature into a world champion on another day.

Even if competitors complete a bout, but suffer head blows, blood clots can quietly and subtly grow and expand into increasingly recognizable symptoms. Catch them while they're young. One is not out of the woods just because a competitor jumps up and down in victory and leaves the arena on his own power.

A very skilled ringside physician friend in Las Vegas witnessed a professional boxer's death in the locker room 30 minutes after a healthy check-up as he exited the ring. Hematomas are deceivingly difficult to diagnose at times.

I treated a female police officer for knee injuries sustained after her police car crashed during a high speed chase. Each visit with me, other medical specialists, and physical therapy confirmed an attractive, alert, polite, and cooperative patient. **Two months** later and only after complaints of forgetfulness and weakness in her trigger finger did x-rays and surgery confirm a small, slowly expanded SUBDURAL HEMATOMA. Her visits with me, internists,

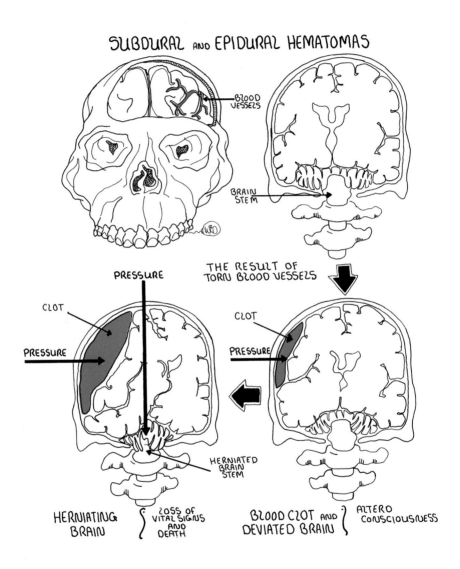

Figure 8-H: Epidural hematoma and subdural hematoma

HEAD INJURY SAFETY GUIDELINES©

CONTACT A PHYSICIAN IF ANY OF THE FOLLOWING OCCUR:

- DIZZINESS OR HEADACHE LASTING OVER ONE HOUR
- INCREASING DROWSINESS
- LOSS OF CONSCIOUSNESS
- MENTAL DISORIENTATION OR CONFUSION
- UNUSUAL OR STRANGE BEHAVIOR
- RESTLESSNESS OR IRRITABILITY
- SEIZURE (CONVULSION)
- BLURRED VISION OR LOSS OF VISION
- REPEATED VOMITING
- BLOOD OR WATERY FLUID FROM EARS OR NOSE
- INABILITY TO CONTROL URINATION OR BOWEL MOVEMENT
- INABILITY TO MOVE AN ARM OR LEG

AVAILABLE THROUGH:
BOXERGENICS™ PRESS, 335 BILLINGSLEY ROAD, CHARLOTTE, NC 28211

1-800-774-MATI (1-800-774-6284)

Figure 8-I: Boxergenics™ Head injury safety guideline chart

and plastic surgeons had failed to establish concerns or visible symptoms. She recovered fully after surgery.

The usual, common warning signs of head injury are provided as a safety net. (Figure 8-I)

I carry copies of this "head sheet" in my doctor kit to athletic events. Without hesitation, I hand these out to any athlete deserving extra attention. Hand-out "head sheets" and enlarged charts are available to display in your locker rooms, training halls, or karate studios. Call Boxergenics™ Press, 1-800-774-6284, to order.

Don't use aspirin or narcotics for headaches occurring after a head injury. Aspirin and possibly non-steroidal anti-inflammatories (NSAID's) might cause greater bleeding and narcotics could mask important symptoms.

SECOND IMPACT SYNDROME

Dr. Robert Cantu, famed neurosurgeon in Boston, author of *Boxing and Medicine,* and past President of the American College of Sports Medicine, has popularized an uncommon but treacherous situation entitled ***Second Impact Syndrome.*** His research and experience have elucidated the underlying wisdom of adequately protecting an athlete from a second successive exposure to head blow. This syndrome occurs soon after a seemingly minor head injury is suffered by an individual who is still experiencing symptoms from a prior concussion. This syndrome, which involves rapid swelling of the brain, has a 50% fatality rate. Seemingly minor head punches to a martial artist or soccer "headings" by a defensive back can prove fatal if either youth had slipped in the shower or fallen off their bike some days prior. HEAD INJURED ATHLETES MUST BE WITHHELD FROM COMPETITION UNTIL AN ADEQUATE SAFETY PERIOD IS SATISFIED. Beware of more than one match in a day, routinely planned in martial arts tournaments.

DEHYDRATION AND HEAD INJURY

Recent, preliminary research suggests that dehydration (weight loss to achieve a body weight class) increases the chance for head injury. Since the brain floats in a buffering layer of spinal fluid, a lowered fluid content might expose the brain surface to uncushioned impact. Recent ringside deaths have been noticeably associated with rapid pre-bout weight loss and restriction of fluids. A loss of 1kg body weight translates into a 1 liter depletion (1 Gallon = 9 Pounds). Performance and safety hinge on a healthy ratio of fat weight and lean body weight. Although elite male athletes train in the 4% - 10% body fat range, the average healthy college man is 13% - 15% body fat. Dehydration is a lousy method to suddenly "make weight. " Dehydration greater than 5% of your total body weight ruins your muscular endurance. In fact, your stamina (aerobic capacity) may decrease with as little as a 2% - 3% loss of body weight due to dehydration. No wonder starved and thirsty athletes lose and get injured!

Replace fluids! Allow plenty of time to rehydrate before competing. Dehydration not only degrades performance and endurance but may predispose to brain injury in contact sports.

NECK INJURY

The cervical spine is quite similarly constructed like its big brother, the low back. It is, however, the weak sister and more delicate. The thick, dense, low back vertebrae were meant to support structural loads, i. e. , carrying bricks and backpacks, loading trucks and trailers. The neck was not designed to be load-bearing as some bridging wrestlers or spearing defensive-backs in football assume. Discs can wear, vertebrae can crush, nerves can be pinched, and spurs can develop. Any of these four possibilities can become reality in the combat arts.

Neck strength is critical for many reasons. A thick, well-stabilized strut of muscles can protect the spine from excessive destabilizing movement at times of impact. Shoulders that seem to blend into the ears will allow the wrestler, judo practitioner, and boxer to diffuse shock-like blows and torquing loads. But, we can only ask so much. Improper training can subtly prove as damaging in the long term as clearly obvious traumatic events. Bridging as an exercise must be practiced in respectful moderation. View bridging as a technique to be learned, not as a safe repetitive exercise. As a high school wrestler in the mid 60's, I joined my more gung-ho teammates in doing bench presses while in the neck bridge position. I would bridge while two wrestlers would hand me a loaded barbell to "rep out" with. The weight would be well over 100 pounds. I expect that we all have matching neck x-rays now to parallel the matching bull necks we proudly possessed then. The neck was never designed to be weight-bearing. Understand your anatomical objectives and realities. With some non-pertinent exceptions, we do not make the vertebrae of a healthy young man stronger by weight training. The focus of your training is, overwhelmingly, to increase muscle mass and strength. We don't have to sacrifice the bones, discs, and joints to challenge the muscles. Forget and avoid axial loading and compression. Great ranges of motion and highly repetitive movements don't have to be performed for gains. **Work the muscle, not the bone.**

How can we do this? Challenge the neck in its more natural and neutral position. Perform short arc movements. Isometrics also effectively apply. Machines like Nautilus are useful. However, limit your range of motion towards the central arcs of movement. Don't take it to extremes. Your muscles will get the message.

Buddy-training is a great exercise tool as long as there are no clowns in the group. Working the neck in the buddy-system, if misused, is a potentially dangerous approach and highly user dependent. An assistant can either use his hands or a towel to resist you through the three arcs described. (Figure 8-J) These are tremendously effective. I taught these to a dedicated workout buddy in college. He and another weight lifter so aggressively trained one day that he starved for the next day or two. His neck muscles were so overworked and extremely sore that he couldn't chew his food or tolerate laughing and coughing the next day. He wasn't injured, just extremely sore in a muscular sense. Go easy at first.

INJURIES

Fractures of the spine do occur in the martial arts, grappling, and wrestling. They are rare in boxing. Martial artists are at risk by direct blows, throws, and falls. It is not so much the bones we worry about, but the delicate spinal cord and nerves that travel through the protective bony canals and outlets. Refer to my section on head injury for proper evacuation of neck injured competitors. Ligamentous tears can render the cervical spine dangerously unstable with the identical neurologic concerns as fracture. Immobilize the cervical spine with a towel if subtle injury is questioned. Initial x-rays may be required followed by additional views with your neck flexed forward and extended backward. Loose vertebrae can be just as dangerous as broken vertebrae. Realize that

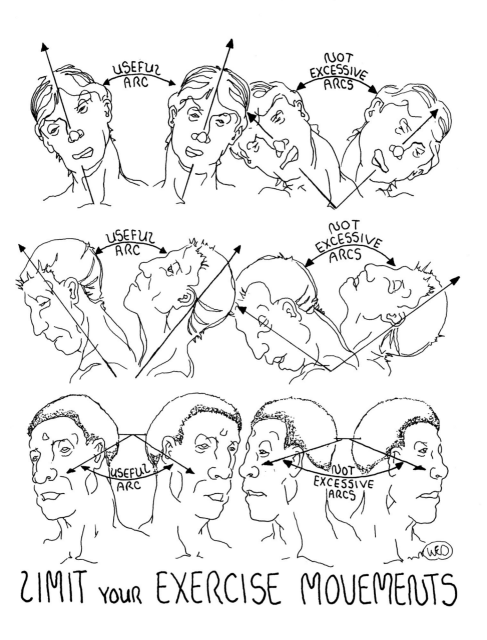

Figure 8-J: Three useful arcs as opposed to three excessive arcs

rather obvious and significant trauma is necessary to cause this type of damage. If you do have any radiation of pain or numbness into your extremities—seek help immediately.

DISCS

Discs are shock absorbers—plain and simple! Too heavy a load and they wear out. A slipped disc, ruptured disc, and bulging disc all mean the same thing, except in degree. Most importantly, is your disc worn and bulging to either a small, medium, or large degree? Larger bulges or free fragments have a greater chance of pushing against a neighboring nerve root or the spinal cord. Because a rather thick ligament strip covers the midline of each disc, the bulges tend to protrude more to the left or right. Therefore, symptoms that travel down an arm and into a hand will more likely cause one-sided symptoms. An arm ache, pins and needles, numbness or weakness in a hand should point fingers back up to the cervical spine. Athletes certainly can injure a cervical disc.

Your doctor's physical exam has the ability to produce a rather accurate estimate of the injury location by "mapping out" your exact areas of complaint. (Figure 8-K)

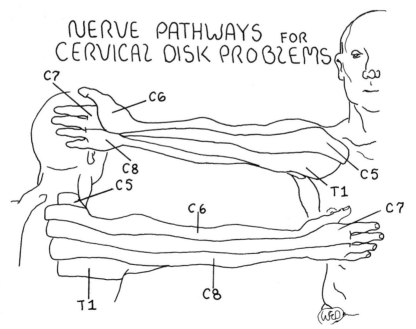

Figure 8-K: Hand and arm chart (nerves that exit from the neck follow a very reproducible pathway)

Each nerve that exits from the neck follows a very reproducible pathway. Your doctor should:

1. Examine neck for range of **movement** and areas of **tenderness**

2. Record biceps and triceps **reflexes**—left and right sides should be symmetric

3. Notice any area of **atrophy** (wasted muscles)

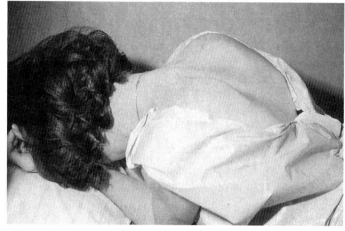

4. Evaluate the symmetry of **strength** in your:
   - Deltoids
   - Biceps
   - Triceps
   - Grip

Figure 8-L: Examination position for levator scapulae syndrome

5. Map out areas of **numbness** or tingling in the arms and hands

6. Place you in the Estwanik "prone and propped" position to isolate **tender tendon insertions** that commonly accompany neck sprains and spasm such as levator scapulae syndrome. (Figure 8-L)

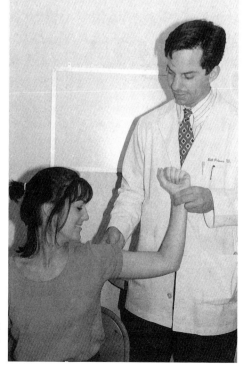

Figure 8-M: Classic examination position useful in evaluation for thoracic outlet syndrome

7. Check your arm **pulses** to be sure that your circulation is not compressed in the upper thorax (thoracic outlet syndrome). Pulses should be checked with your arm in the 90° - 90° position and be calculated both with head-turning and breath-holding. (Figure 8-M)

If an injured disc is diagnosed, either a surgical or non-surgical course of treatment is necessary. An MRI (magnetic resonance imaging) will precisely localize the injured tissues. This imaging study will also define the magnitude of the injury so that your chances for non-surgical options are better calculated.

A conservative treatment plan includes:

- Rest
- Neck supports
- Anti-inflammatories
- Pain pills
- Traction
- Chiropractic
- Ice
- TENS unit
- Injections to areas of tendonitis
- Physical therapy modalities (ultrasound/muscle stimulation/cortisone phonophoresis)
- Stretches, muscle exercises, ranges of motion—all at later stages

Many disc ruptures will slowly heal and not require surgical removal. Maintain close supervision by a specialist. (See my explanation of disc rupture under lumbar spine). I once supervised the healing of a full blown cervical disc rupture in Ric Flair, a very well-known professional wrestler. This massively muscled athlete had once successfully competed as a power lifter. His classic symptoms of neck pain, numbness traveling into his fingers, and arm weakness slowly resolved with his extremely dedicated attention to conservative treatment. At one point he was unable to bench press 135 pounds because of an affected and weakened triceps muscle. He has fully recovered and for the past seven years has triumphantly performed on televised, super-show, pay-per-view events. He did not require surgery.

FACET INJURY (Figure 8-N)

Facets are the small, shingled, paired joints that glide ever-so-slightly as one moves their neck. They can become sprained or wear-out just like any larger joint such as the knee, elbow, or hip. It is difficult to view them precisely on x-rays, but obvious degeneration can be visualized. Many times, a "sprained" neck will actually be caused by a facet that is traumatized. Many

of those same conservative treatment options listed for disc injuries will produce a cure.

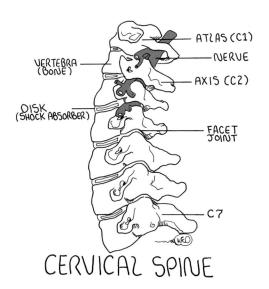

Figure 8-N: C-spine

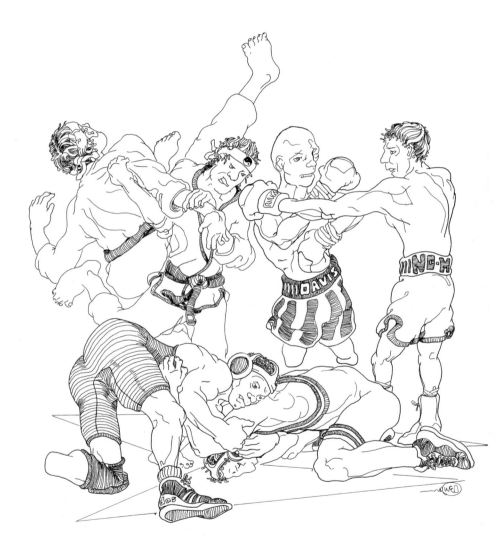

Chapter 9

Chokes and Joint Locks

In preparing for a trip, what details must you consider in making your plans? If attending an athletic event what gear do you pack? If a moderately distant city is our destination, do we drive or fly? Many factors must e analyzed in arriving at our answer. Is flying safe? Supposedly, mile per nile, flying is safer, but other factors must be considered. What airline are you sing? Who is your pilot? How much experience does he have? How many rips (amount of exposure) will you travel as a passenger? A similar array of onsiderations should apply to your practice of the martial arts and other comat arts. Certain techniques require a realistic assessment of their safety ecords and a review of proper utilization.

The rise in popularity of submision and Reality ighting (Figure -A) has been riven to unpreedented public wareness by the Jltimate Fighting Championships, Vorld Combat Championships,

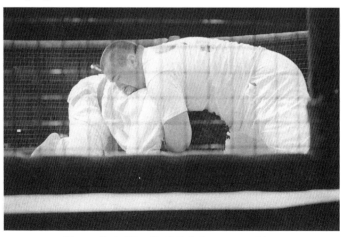

Figure 9-A: "Reality" fighting competition

and Battlecade Extreme Fighting events. Having served as ringside physician and behind-the-scenes medical event coordinator for many of these events prompted me to evaluate the injuries and review the predominant ways of winning. (Figure 9-B)

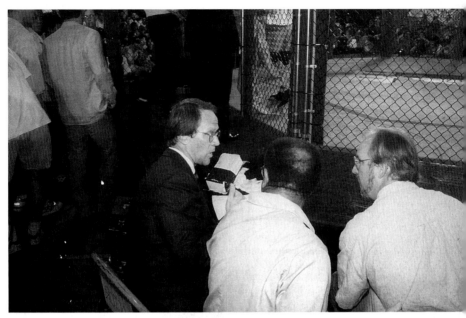

Figure 9-B: Dr. Estwanik as ringside physician during "Reality" fighting bouts.

The internationally acclaimed Gracie jiu-jitsu family has revolutionized the martial arts world. In the recent past, one's height of acclaim paralleled the height of one's kick. The showy, spinning crescent kicks sold videos and from page placement in prominent martial arts magazines. However, a great revolution in technique has occurred. Now, we all know "it ends on the ground." The most popular "finishing" moves now either involve a joint lock or a choke that forces an opponent's submission. A joint lock can be defined as forcefully holding any joint in a position that creates an unnatural painful stress on that joint. Directions of applied force can vary tremendously for any given joint. Each joint is cursed with its idiosyncrasies. Ligaments and the joint capsule contain plentiful nerve fibers and ordinarily signal a joint's awareness of non-anatomic posturing. These nerve fibers most definitely shout during submission hold. A skilled competitor can exert just enough force and unwant

:d angulation to gain a win without exceeding the fine line that crosses into nflicting gross deformity and injury.

Most wrist locks pressure the wrist into excessive flexion, i.e., fingers owards palm (the "come along"), although the pain-producing "Cogie" :stablishes lines of pressure along the thumb-side. Elbow locks routinely lrive this joint into very unnatural hyperextension (too straight). Ankle locks ;ain the attention of the loser when his foot and ankle are involuntarily plan-ar flexed.

CHOKE

A choke (shime-waza in judo) can be lefined as a temporary compression of :ither the airway or the vascular supply >f the brain. Each of these mechanisms ıltimately robs the brain of necessary >xygen, creating unconsciousness. A >roperly applied choke hold precipi-ates a 10 - 20 second unconscious peri->d followed by rapid complete recov-ry. (Figure 9-C)

Law enforcement agencies consider he chokehold a reasonably safe tech-ıique for controlling violent criminals vithout the additional use of weapons lthough many agencies disallow its ıse. Studies have failed to confirm a port fatality by choke since the found-

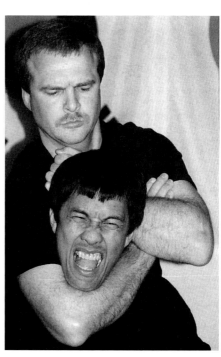

Figure 9-C: Choke hold

ıg of judo by Professor Jigoro Kano over 100 years ago. A 12 year analysis >f world class judo events yielded 2,198 scoring techniques where the choke ıad been applied 4.4% of the time (97 chokes) and no fatalities were record-d. Unfortunately, some non-sport fatal consequences have been reported by)r. Karl Koiwai in the 1987 *Journal of Forensic Sciences*. He specifically valuated 14 alleged deaths from chokes applied to criminals by law enforce-nent officers. As one would expect, most decedents were confirmed drug .busers at their time of death.

A properly ("executed") applied choke-out to the critical area of the neck creates unconsciousness in about 10 seconds. Assuming that this pressure is released in a timely fashion, the "chokee" regains consciousness in about 10 to 20 seconds. Prolonged or excessive pressure spells trouble for both the victim and the choker (now a "legal target"). **All pressure must cease when the opponent submits or goes limp.** What kind of pressure is required? I can't give a practical answer but studies suggest 250 - 300mm Hg. These numbers do translate into a lady possessing the capability of incapacitating (not decapitating) a man twice her size.

The anatomical basis for an effective choke has been studied by Dr. Koiwai in his 1987 article. The superior carotid triangle is an area outlined by the jaw and neck muscles. (Figure 9-D) Obviously, they are paired into identical left and right sides. For important practical application, this target triangle occupies the upper end of the front neck muscles, just below the jaw line. The muscles themselves are not important. Their significance relates to the vital structures that pass through this triangular anatomic landmark. Lots of good stuff calls this area home. Within this triangle is the:

STRUCTURE	FUNCTION
1. Carotid Artery	Main source of blood to the brain
2. Carotid Bodies	Monitor oxygen in blood to the brain, regulating heart rate
3. Internal Jugular Vein	Major vein draining blood from the head
4. Vagus Nerve	Slows breathing and heart rate; affects voice, stomach, and swallowing
5. Recurrent Laryngeal Nerve	Intrinsic muscles of larynx (voice box)
6. Cervical Sympathetic Trunk	Nerves that increase breathing, heart rate, use of blood sugar

Hence, the choke deactivates-activates a scary number of bodily reactions. **Unconsciousness** is related to the lack of oxygen-carrying blood reaching the brain. A slowed heart rate, constricted pupils, and low blood pressure occur secondary to stimulation of the vagus nerve. **Shock** (slow heart rate and low blood pressure) can be due to pressure on the carotid sinus. **Hormonal response** with the drastic release of serum cortisone (17-ketosteroids) can last for six to eight hours. **Minor convulsions** may be present during the uncon-

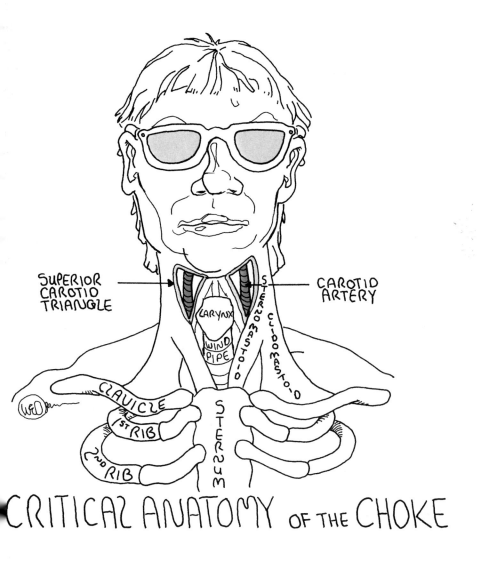

CRITICAL ANATOMY OF THE CHOKE

Figure 9-D: The vulnerable superior carotid triangle

scious state. One may not observe this visually, but brain seizures can be recorded by EEG. They apparently cease upon awakening.

A 1991 article by Rodriguez et al in *The Journal of Sports Medicine and Physical Fitness* analyzed EEG studies on 10 choke-out volunteers. Although their EEG's went bonkers during the actual test period of their unconsciousness, the ten experienced judo subjects possessed normal pre-test baseline studies suggesting no long term consequences. Abnormal EEG (brain wave patterns did appear 10 seconds after the choke began and persisted for 5 to 6 seconds before the EEG tracing gradually returned to normal 15 seconds after the loss of consciousness. Their conclusion suggested no evidence of chronic brain deficits in martial artists after cautious exposure to being choked. Boxers, in contrast, have exhibited permanent resting EEG changes after exposure to excessive head blows over a prolonged pro career.

Another 1991 article by Owens et al in *The Journal of Sports Medicine and Physical Fitness* did highlight a single individual believed to have suffered long term brain injury from choke-outs. This 33 year old with international expertise, who suffered a left-sided stroke and confirmed memory disturbance blamed his judo participation as the cause of his problems.

CHOKE REVIVAL

After a choke-out has occurred, how does one assist and revive the subject? Many wive's tales exist, unfounded in any scientific basis. At a recent late night, post-karate tournament meal, I heard all forms and fashions of treatment recommendations from our "round table" discussions—"set them up and knee them in the spine three times," "slap their face," and "rub their neck," were voiced methods. Every opinion was overshadowed by a questioning "I don't know, but this is what I heard" viewpoint. I need to simplify the treatment concepts. As explained earlier, a vascular choke does just what it says ... it robs the brain of blood and oxygen. We pass out because an insufficient supply of blood transported oxygen fails to circulate into our brain cells. Either direct pressure on arteries or blood pressure-lowering reflexes are directly responsible for the deficiency.

Recovery is exclusively related to a timely restoration of oxygen to the brain. Be absolutely certain that the "victim" is lying perfectly flat on the ground, face up. Water doesn't run uphill very well. Blood doesn't run uphill o the brain efficiently. Don't sit the person up. If he is flat, oxygen-rich blood an more easily supply the deprived brain cells. A great percentage of our total lood volume dwells in our legs. If you also elevate the victims legs, many xtra pints of blood will be dumped towards the head, to accelerate recovery. \ related scenario was brilliantly, elucidated by my fantastically humorous nedical school professor of pathology. Dr. Pritchard emphatically shared his ;reatest nightmare with us—fainting in a telephone booth, unable to fall down. Iis vivid physiologic fear simplified my understanding of fainting and the orrect sequence of revival.

The normal sequence of falling to the ground as one faints follows a design f nature. Blood supply recirculates to restore alertness, open eyes, and reor- anize thoughts. Don't abandon basics to stoke the fires of myth just because ainting was induced by "oriental" methods. It's all the same. Retreat to basics. ome acupuncture, acupressure points when stimulated may assist recovery. am open-minded and aware that I am leaving "the door cracked open" when naking this statement. However, don't exclude the basics of physiology.

1. Supine position.

2. Airway cleared by chin elevation.

3. Elevation of the legs.

4. If recovery of spontaneous breathing and pulse don't return within 20 to 40 seconds, assume problems.

5. Re-evaluate the A, B, C, D'S of resuscitation—airway, breathing, circu- lation.

I have personally witnessed the choke applied voluntarily during demon- trations, as well as applied during true competitions. Famous tournament ghter John Perretti, director of Battlecade Extreme Fighting, demonstrated is technique of choke revival on the carpeted floor of the penthouse suite that e utilized as "command module" for the tournament. Before my eyes a choke as applied until the very casually volunteering "chokee" went limp at 8 sec- nds. Highly athletic, action actor, ring announcer, and former American Glad- ttor star, Viper (Scott Berlinger), was instantaneously and totally revived by narp fingertip pressure to his supraclavicular area. Both instructors mentioned witnessing suspect revival methods whereby the victim is kneed between hi shoulder blades. Much quality research needs to be completed. Be wary!

Just as I earlier assessed the safety of flying, one must analyze the spars data on the choke-out. Like flying, the risks are very small with any one iso lated choke maneuver. But, who is our "pilot" and how experienced is he? Th person applying the choke must know what he is doing. Excessive pressur can damage surrounding structures such as our windpipe (trachea) or injur our spinal column. A choke applied for too great a time period can rob ou brain of essential oxygen, causing permanently damaged brain cells. Th autopsy reports on 14 criminals, who died in conflicts with an arresting offi cer, confirmed that they succumbed to overzealous choke forces. To be fai these drug-crazed criminals would have been alternatively and fatally sub dued by gunfire had the hand-to-hand combat not prevailed. However, a prac ticed and skilled master would understand the minimum force necessary t accomplish his intent. Every martial artist must be keenly learned in ever detail of finesse.

Who supervises? In any competitive situation, the overseeing refere coach, or instructor must supply constant vigilance. A poorly maintained plan will crash. A poorly maintained training session or tournament will crash.

The literature has already supplied an unfortunate case history of a partic ipant who was choked-out one too many times. The more you fly, the great risk you assume. Don't take this blood and oxygen robbing maneuver to lightly. "Frequent flyers" are at risk!

Chapter 10

Facial

Accumulated blows to the face and orbital area can create macabre swelling for the initial day or two post bout. Most certainly, a ringside or sports physician should be consulted to confirm that the swelling is superficial only and that no deep structures were compromised. Figure 10-A) Many boxers will wear sunglasses to hide their losses. While boxing the Russians, one of our boxers, Steve, took quite a beating. He was depressed, angry, frustrated, and embarrassed. He perked up from his slumped position on the team bus when one "well meaning" teammate, named Riddick Bowe, offered a seemingly encouraging explanation for his humiliating defeat. "Your opponent was cheating! I saw it! I saw it!" Steve grew several inches taller as comfort was tantalizingly dangled before his glasses-covered, grotesquely swollen, raccoon eyes. "He had something **on** his gloves. He had something **all over** his gloves!" A glint of ego-

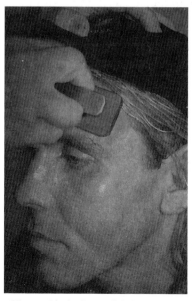

Figure 10-A: Superficial swelling

strengthening hope sat him up straighter yet. "What was it?" petitioned Steve. With all on the bus now tuned into the mystery, Riddick looked right through Steve's dark glasses and responded—"Your face!" Riddick will never, ever be hired as our team's sports psychologist. It would be better that we turn his mischievous humor on our enemy.

CUTS

After a bout is completed, winners and losers must have their wounds and injuries evaluated. USA Boxing requires that all boxers cooperate with a post-bout exam. More then once, I have encountered a poor loser (the winners are graciously cooperative) who refuses to allow an exam. One malcontent even "verbally" punched me with some four-letter words as I attempted my ringside obligations. No problem handling that situation—"Don't get mad, just get even." I defensively rationalized that since this defeated fighter didn't possess the "good sense" to be examined, a head injury must have occurred. All head injuries receive an automatic 30 day suspension. Guess how rapidly the boxer was hauled back by his coach for an exam? The suspension remained. The word quickly spread that this doctor takes his duties seriously and that cooperation with the rules is most compatible with future opportunities to compete. The post-bout evaluation promotes a thorough assessment of injuries and their consequences.

As a ringside physician I do recommend stoppage of a bout if the competitor is taking a beating. Head blows are scary and dramatically elevate my powers of observation to "hyper alert" monitoring status. My tolerance for an unsteady gait or loss of defensive skills is best described as a "short fuse." The usual reaction from the boxer and his coach are **briefly** a "why did you stop it, Doc?" attitude. Shortly thereafter, I am routinely rewarded by a thankfully reassuring "good call, Doc" remark from that same pair. Yet, if a cut appears (however small or however minor) there is a consensus opinion to "don't let it go on too long." A boxer can be getting his brains beat out, yet the sight of blood from a minor facial laceration brings echoing cries like "he's been cut man!"—signals of doom and gloom! It doesn't make sense to me! I can't figure it out! Don't ask me why! Questioning thoughts about folklore circle through my mind as I sit at ringside observing a coach's fears of bleeding while simultaneous head blows are mounting steadily. Facial cuts are poorly under stood by the boxing and fighting community. Cuts are readily fixable if understood properly, while head injuries are very unforgiving and dangerous.

Dr. Robert Voy, noted ringside physician of Las Vegas, Nevada, in *The Ringside Physician's Certification Manual* by USA Boxing, clearly classifies the cuts of a boxer (fighter). (Figure 10-B)

- Cuts in area "A" rarely lead to long term disability, do not endanger vision, nor damage significant underlying structures.

- However, cuts "B" (supraorbital nerve) or "C" in the area of the infraorbital nerve and nasal lacrimal duct may indicate that a bout be stopped.

- Cuts "D" in the upper eyelid can endanger the tarsal plate.

- Vertical cuts "E" through the border of the lip create the potential for further tearing.

- Cuts "F" near the bridge of the nose require a doctor to certify that an underlying open nasal fracture or injury to the bony orbit surrounding the eye does not exist.

- Cuts localized near the medial aspect of the eye (near the bridge of the nose) are dangerous because the tear (lacrimal) duct lies very close to the skin surface. This area should be sutured by experts only as a deep suture

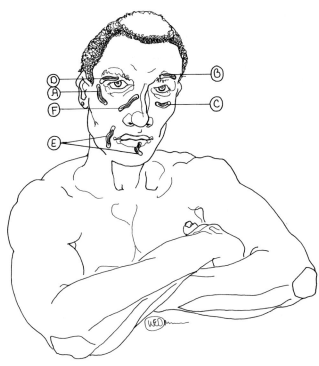

Figure 10-B: Cuts of a fighter

could tie-off this duct requiring further extensive reconstructive surgeries. A competitor in Battlecade Extreme Fighting suffered such an injury from a left hook punch. Because his cut was rather small, we elected not to chance a suture in this location.

Plentiful misunderstanding exists! The ringside doctor must sort out minor from major injuries. Needless over-reaction or dangerous under-reaction can sway the action and outcome of a bout. Experienced ringside physicians are a rare commodity but USA Boxing has initiated a program that provides ringside physician certification. I have personally designed an annual Ringside Physician's Course held in conjunction with USA Boxing's National Championships hosted at the Olympic Training Center, Colorado Springs, Colorado.

Cuts to the face of a combatant are not at all similar to lacerations from a sharp object like a knife or surgical scalpel. You should understand the mechanics of these facial cuts as similar to those of a gunshot with its little entrance wound but large internal cavitation. (Figure 10-C)

The typical laceration by a sharp object is an outside insult that is extended inward to the underlying tissues. The "punched" facial

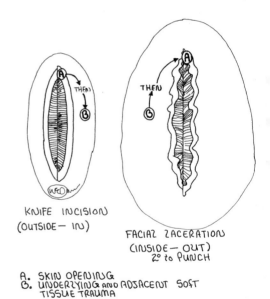

KNIFE INCISION
(OUTSIDE — IN)

FACIAL LACERATION
(INSIDE — OUT)
2° to PUNCH

A. SKIN OPENING
B. UNDERLYING and ADJACENT SOFT
TISSUE TRAUMA

Figure 10-C: Mechanics of cuts

cut represents a skin-bursting injury that begins with deeply damaged tissues. Believe it or not, the cut actually begins against the bone as the skin is forced against those underlying bony ridges. Boxer's cuts are "inside-out" cuts. The bones of the face are the "sharp" objects that cause the skin to finally split or explode open externally. Thus, most of the damage is truly dealt to the subcutaneous tissues rather than misleadingly apparent on the skin surface. What fans recognize as a "cut" is only the tip of the iceberg.

The basics of **cuts in boxers-fighters** are as follows:

1. Don't freak out at a minor cut. A little red blood goes a long way. The face is a very vascular area.

2. Recognize lacerations that might become dangerous because of their proximity to underlying important structures.

3. Understand that more tissue is damaged deep to the skin than is first evident. Understand that tissues deep to the skin are more extensively damaged than superficially evident, i.e., these cuts are inside-out injuries.

4. A sutured wound heals faster and stronger than a comparable non-repaired wound.

5. The application of buried subcutaneous sutures in combination with visible skin sutures is the superior method of closure in deeper cuts.

One of our boxers was cut during a recent bout against England hosted at their traditional competition site, the exquisite London Hilton. For 33 years, a private Jewish businessman's organization has annually raised hundreds of thousands of dollars during the winter holiday season in support of orphanages. A boxing ring visually dominated the center of the main ballroom. Tuxedos and Bentleys quite noticeably, yet respectfully, clashed with the sweat and blood. Our experienced 145-pounder, Mike, sustained a noticeably bloody, but very superficial cut under his left eye during the second round. His cut characteristics typified the scenario of healing tissues. My evaluation after his bout confirmed a very superficial, ragged, splitting of skin. The previously injured skin of this experienced boxer raggedly spread open rather than simply cut. Multiple prior punches to this same prominent cheek bone degraded his skin into a soft, thin, flimsy tissue. His opponent's blow merely split the skin as if over-stretched into the appearance of a fine fissure on the skin of an over-ripe tomato. No sutures were required for this minor gap. Most of the trauma and swelling came from deep. His skin had merely been forcefully stretched and crushed again over the high ridges of his classic Anglo-Saxon face. His many bouts of scar production are not a satisfactory substitute for real, natural skin, as each behaves differently.

Many boxers are shaken up by the thought of being sutured. "The cut can't be that bad" they claim. I patiently explain that the judicious suturing of an appropriate facial cut offers not only the most rapid return to competition but the best assurance against a reopening during future bouts. A "better quality" scar results when the edges are brought into direct contact. If left unsutured and gaping, the void must slowly fill-in with substitute scar, a weak secondary putty. In addition, a significantly deep cut will

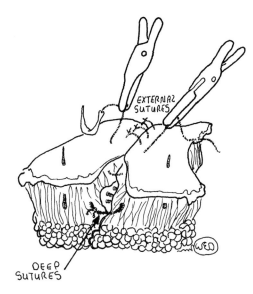

Figure 10-D: Deeper stitches support an improved healing wound

heal more efficiently if its deeper portions are additionally supported by an absorbable stitch. The deeper stitches: (Figure 10-D)

1. close the deep gap so that fluid or hematoma won't develop.

2. bring the deeper tissues in proximity to strengthen the wound and decrease the need for scar to fill the void.

3. decrease tension on the visible skin sutures so that a prettier scar results

Wound healing time occupies many more weeks than one would guess. In fact, it has been estimated that even if a wound is repaired, it takes three months just to attain 60% of pre-injury strength. Boxing doctor and plastic surgeon, Steve Goodman, M.D., of Schenectady, New York, estimates wound strength as follows:

30 Days - 20% Strength

60 Days - 50% Strength

1 Year   - 80% Strength

A scar is never as strong as normal tissue. I have explained this line of reasoning so often to competitors that I have rationalized that in order to save words, it is easier to write a book.

HEADGEAR

Headgear with cheek protection can really minimize the incidence of cuts. (Figure 10-E) In 1981, 1982, and 1983, when I covered USA Boxing National Championships before their mandatory headgear rules, lacerations were plentiful. We would expect so many cuts during tournaments that we actually designated "suture rooms" within each tournament facility. Essentially, a physician was assigned to this room while the other docs covered the rings. Duties were rotated. Now that headgear is mandated for amateurs, cuts are a rarity. Professional boxing and martial arts can well profit from this statistic. Cauliflower ears have also been drastically reduced in boxers because of head protection.

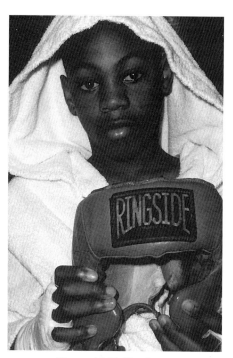

Figure 10-E: Headgear

MOUTH GUARDS

Proper use and fit of mouth guards can:

1. Limit lacerations of the cheek and lips

2. Protect the teeth

3. Prevent jaw fractures

4. Limit tongue lacerations

5. Possibly decrease the forces of brain concussion as these forces are dissipated and better absorbed

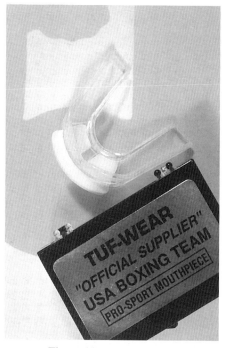

Figure 10-F: Mouthpiece

6. Protect the temporomandibular joints (TMJ's) from impaction and future arthritic change

Only the use of a custom fit mouthpiece is acceptable when involved in combat sports. (Figure 10-F)

ORBITAL

Broken bones around the orbit (eye socket) can, "as you see," carry dangerous complications. The danger lies not so much in the actual bony structure being injured but its close proximity to major delicate structures of the eye. Just as real estate consultants classically stress "location, location, location" as their three most important considerations, the gravity of facial injury is likewise determined by the critical location of adjacent structures. Place the palm of your hand directly over your eye. Unless, you are hyperthyroid, with bulging eyeballs, your palm doesn't contact your eye but rests upon natural bony buttresses. Blows to the eye region are initially absorbed by these bones thus preserving our vision. It most usually takes an ungloved finger or the thumb of a boxing glove to funnel pressure onto the globe. The recent adoption of thumbless or thumb-attached boxing gloves has considerably decreased eye injury. Once again, hi-tech equipment design has made a sport safer. The prominence of these bony ridges does, however, facilitate cuts and fractures. Our prior chapter explained how boxer's cuts occur as the bony ridges cut adjacent skin compressed against it by a fist. These cuts are best understood as **inside-out.**

Just several months ago I was ringside physician at a national championship for 17 year olds. I don't specifically remember caring for Andre at ringside but 18 hours after his bout he approached me with a bizarre complaint. At that time I was the official physician assigned by the Olympic Committee for coverage of our Winter Olympic Training Center in Lake Placid, New York. Each volunteer physician lives on-site, day and night, for two weeks providing coverage for camps, competitions, and daily care for the elite athletes residing in house. The boxing tournament was one of many sports activities scheduled. I was running from bobsledding to speed-skating to free-style ski jump to luge to boxing. Andre's appearance and story did catch my attention. He had boxed the previous evening. His immediate post-bout exam and a relaxed evening spent with his teammates signaled no war wounds except for the hurt of his disappointing defeat. Breakfast and lunch proved paradise to an athlete who had been sacrificing teenage food binges in his efforts to make weight. Just after lunch he blew his nose and immediately felt his eye bulge as it became a toy balloon pressurized with helium. Still, there was no pain, only a grotesquely puffy, spongy eye. With the cafeteria immediately across a hall-way from the sportsmedicine center, he quickly sprinted into our clinic. (Figure 10-G)

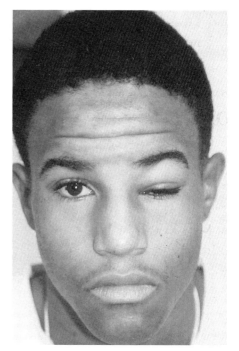

Figure 10-G: Andre's eye bulge

Seeing is believing! Further examination failed to produce additional findings. His nose and bony ridges about the eye demonstrated no tenderness. Visual checks confirmed excellent eye sight and eye movement. In these circumstances one would evaluate for:

1. Local tenderness

2. Pupil size and its reaction to light

3. Eye movement

4. Ability to read printed material

5. Ability to see objects overhead, low, and to the far right and left (visual fields)

6. Double vision

7. Blood in the anterior chamber (area of the eye just in front of the pigmented iris)—hyphema

8. Possible tears of the retina by use of a medical instrument (ophthalmoscope)

That same afternoon he was referred to an eye, ear, nose, and throat specialist who confirmed the only injury that could be responsible for this classic presentation. A punch to the bones of his medial orbit had caused distortion and created a pin-point defect in the very thin bony wall that separates the eye from the nose and its sinus cavities. The increased pressure from blowing his nose forced air through the defective ethmoid sinus's (lamina papyracea) cribriform plate wall and into the eye socket. (Figure 10-H) Because his actual bone defect was so minor, no special care was needed—only time (6-8 weeks) However, antibiotics were a necessity as germs from the nasal sinuses could easily be carried into the sterile eye re

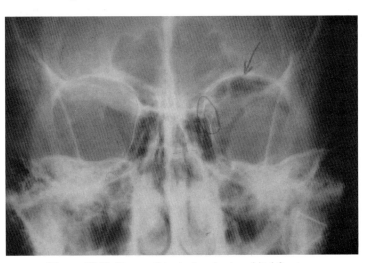

Figure 10-H: X-ray of Andre's minute orbital fracture

gion with disastrous consequences. This young man **and his coach** were given strict orders to be certain he obtained a follow-up consult with an ENT specialist upon returning home.

A more frequent and dangerous fracture is aptly termed a "blow-out" fracture of the orbital floor. The most usual symptoms of this defect would include

1. An interference with upward gaze

2. Enophthalmos (the entire eyeball sinking inward towards the skull)

3. Double vision

Although our patient Andre demonstrated unusual manifestations from a defect on the inner wall of the orbit, the floor of the orbit is commonly injured by direct punches to the face. If the floor of the orbit is shattered, the eyeball and its muscles can drop downward and its movements "tied up." When both eyes can't move in unison with a coordinated effort, double vision results. One eye aims one way, and the other eye another. This jokingly reminds me of the proverbial ugly date from Hell with "blue" eyes—one blew this way and one blew that way. Even if the difference of eye control is slight, two images are seen. Which opponent does the boxer now punch? Surgical reconstruction is necessary to restore vision.

CHEEK BONE

The zygomatic bone is our "cheek bone." A good, strong left hook, elbow, head-butt, or knee to the side of the face can "stove in" this area—the cheek would appear flat. In addition to localized pain the athlete would exhibit "trismus"—a painful difficulty in fully opening and closing the jaw since these associated muscles are compressed by the injury. Surgical reconstruction is necessary not only for cosmesis, but to prevent problems with opening-closing the jaw.

JAW

A broken jaw—mandible—is a definite indication to stop a bout and seek medical care. One can evaluate an injured player in several ways. See if she can open her mouth. Feel if any teeth appear loose. Ask if the individual's "bite" seems normal to them when they clamp their jaw together. Test for tenderness by having them slowly bite down on a wooden popsicle stick (a non-tooth chipping material). Obtain x-rays. While I was serving as ringside physician for the semi-finals of our National Championships (USA Boxing), our second ranked, 165 pound boxer complained of jaw and tooth pain. He had won his bout and not signaled his coach or doctor that something was abnormal during the third round. He was definitely one tough young man. My exam revealed gross movement of three adjacent front teeth on his lower jaw. X-rays demonstrated the teeth to be loose because his jaw bone (mandible) had broken and the three attached teeth were moving together at the actual fracture site. His jaw was repaired by wiring his teeth together but days later, Steve assured me that he couldn't wait to resume training. Fractures of the lower jaw or facial bones adjacent to our upper teeth can sometimes be treated and stabilized by wiring the teeth together rather than operating directly upon the fracture site itself.

CAULIFLOWER EAR

"Wrestler's ear," "Boxer's ear" are common terms that prove self-explanatory. A picture is worth 1,000 words. (Figure 10-I) Few, however, understand why such an injury persists. Our ears (and nose) are stiffened by multi-layered cartilage that lies between the layers of skin. Compare this human anatomy to the multi-layered rock—mica. A glancing blow shears the layers of mica (splits the layer of cartilage) and allows blood to accumulate between layers. This blood soon clots and that clot permanently forms a deforming bulge. Unless this fresh clot is aspirated with a needle, the adjacent layers won't adhere together again and get filled with scar. Be

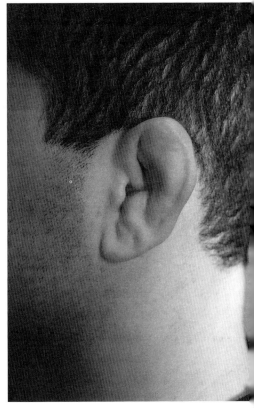

Figure 10-I: Cauliflower ear of master Brazilian jiu-jitsu expert (Ralph Gracie)

sure this procedure is performed only under the strictest of **sterile technique**. Once the hematoma is pulled out by a syringe—a firm pressure bandage must be applied to close the dead space and prevent reaccumulation of bleeding. Once the layers stick back together, the gross deformity is banished.

There are several techniques to prevent the return of this clot:

1. Cotton soaked in Collodion will harden and form a mini-cast. Extra layers of cotton sponges placed behind and in front of the ear can be held in place by a turban-like bandage wrapped about the head. It looks weird but must be worn for several days. Self-conscious teenagers prefer to cut classes while dressed so oddly.

2. Sometimes the nose-clips worn when swimming can be modified to compress these ear tissues. Pad safely to prevent secondary tissue necrosis from pressure.

3. Large hematomas may require that a suture is placed all the way through the ear tissues. Tying this stitch over cotton pads holds the layers firmly compressed—suggested only for difficult injuries.

Cauliflower ear is preventable nowadays. Headgear is a must. There is very little excuse for a high school wrestler wearing deformed ears. Boxers rarely live with these injuries now that headgear is required for amateurs.

EARDRUM RUPTURES

A "slapping" punch (with the hand open) even with headgear in place, imparts a vacuum phenomenon to the ear. This concussive effect tears ("ruptures") the eardrum. Pain is certainly a factor and poor hearing accompanies this tear. I do see this injury with some regularity. Using headgear doesn't cancel the powerful pressure created from a slap.

I routinely test a boxer's hearing by rubbing my fingertips together several inches from each ear. I don't ask "Can you hear this?" since an automatic "yes" only confirms that a boxer will say "yes" in order to pass the test. Rather the game goes as follows—"Tell me **when** you hear my fingers rubbing together near **each** ear." A delay means that I pull an otoscope out of my doctor's kit and actually peer into each ear as I visibly inspect the circular eardrum for defects.

I don't allow a competitor with a rupture to compete for two reasons:

1. We don't want to interfere with nature's healing process. Usually cells will re-grow over the defect just as outreaching grass can fill-in bare spots within our lawn. If the tear and gap isn't too large, our bodies can manage a repair. We don't want to impede the progress of these cells and necessitate a surgery.

2. With a hole present, our delicate middle ear bones—the hammer, anvil, and stirrup—are exposed to the micro evils of the outside world—germs. Avoid water splashing into that ear while showering. No swimming. Don't put drops in your ear. An **oral** antibiotic should be initially prescribed. Apply cotton daily to your ear to protect from outside contamination.

Seek clearance from an ear, nose, throat specialist to confirm good healing and good hearing. Remember, pain pills, cotton ear plug, and oral antibiotics are the initial steps in treatment.

NOSE BLEEDS (EPISTAXIS)

Nothing so prominently hangs out there for all the world to punch as our nose. Even minor playground disputes leave teachers applying first-aid to the loser's seemingly endless flow of blood. There are some "tricks of the trade"— more specifically hints for stopping bleeding, not starting it. First, an anatomy lesson is necessary for understanding. (Figure 10-J)

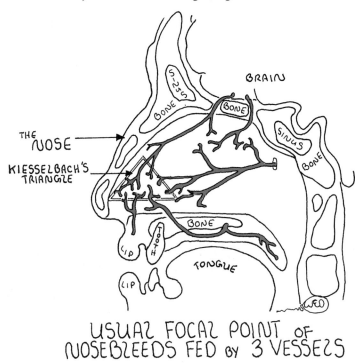

Figure 10-J: Anatomy of nose bleeds

Most don't realize that a great portion of their nose is composed of cartilage and not bone. Use thumb and index finger to grip your nose and wiggle the tip. Only the area close to your skull is firm, fixed bone. Kiesselbach's plexus is a very vascular concentration of vessels prominently occupying the septum dividing your nasal passages into left and right nostrils. The typical nose bleed arises from these superficial blood vessels on either side of the septum. A simple nose bleed can be effectively controlled by pinching the nostrils with thumb and index finger. Usually one minute of pressure between rounds establishes control of the free flow of blood. Some bleeding might occur in the following round if the nose is re-traumatized, but I prefer to allow the boxer's corner personnel to handle this situation one round at a time. Minor problems respond well to this menu. **Importantly**—tip the head slightly forward with chin toward chest rather than chin towards ceiling or by lying down. The latter two incorrect positions only allow the blood to trickle down your throat, lessening pressure that clots the injury site. **REMEMBER: NOSTRILS PINCHED AND HEAD TIPPED SLIGHTLY DOWNWARD.** Don't blow your nose soon thereafter to clear your breathing! This activity only removes the clot and restarts the corked bleeding site. On more than one unhappy occasion my shirt has been terminally polka-dotted with spattered blood as I entered the ring to evaluate a nosebleed. Now, a forceful command—"Do not blow your nose" precedes my appearance at the summit of the steps. In professional hands, a cigarette-shaped dental packing or cotton swab soaked in adrenaline can quickly stop most routine nasal bleeding.

If there is rather severe pain from gripping one's nose, uncontrolled bleeding, or deformity, assume that a nose is broken. If a boxer winces as I pinch his nose during an exam at ringside, a fracture is suspected. I, obviously, don't allow a martial artist or boxer to continue if nasal fracture is suspected. A routine nose bleed doesn't cause much localized pain. I shine a flashlight onto the back

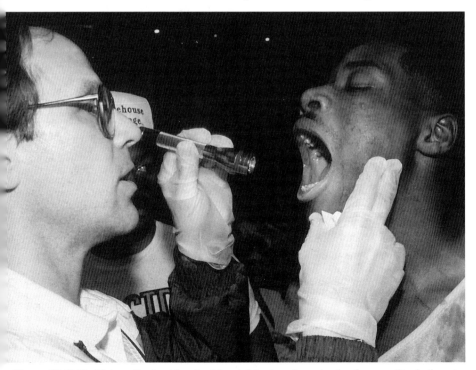

Figure 10-K:Dr. Estwanik checking for blood dripping down back of competitor's throat.

of a competitor's throat to be certain that blood is not dripping down, as this flow suggests excessive or dangerous bleeding. (Figure 10-K) If gazing into the nose reveals a pressurized collection of blood under the mucosal lining on either side of the nasal septum, a septal hematoma is present. This "blueberry" appearing hematoma needs drainage by a doctor in order to avoid pressure necrosis to the nasal septum. See a (ear, nose, throat) specialist if you suspect this problem. A broken nose will assuredly drain the fight out of a fighter. Obtain x-rays for confirmation. (Figure 10-L and Figure 10-M) A nose is usually "set" three to five

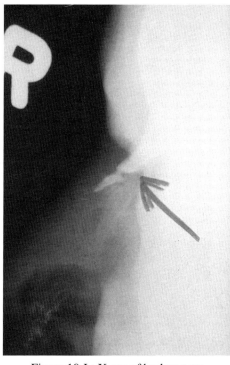

Figure 10-L: X-ray of broken nose

days after injury, but soon thereafter fitness training, not competing, is allowed. Sometimes an active boxer with repeated nose injury will request cosmetic nasal surgery, but we recommend this only after his career has ended. One eventually "fixes" a nose because healthy breathing is chronically impaired. Improper humidification of our inhaled air leads to health problems. Surgery is recommended for more reasons than just cosmesis.

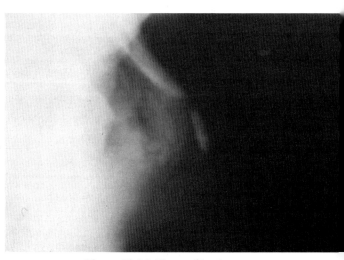

Figure 10-M: X-ray of broken nose

Chapter 11

Eye Trauma

A study of professional boxers in New York state by Dr. Vincent Giovanazzo of Manhattan confirmed that 66% of these competitors suffered from a documentable eye injury. This specialized ophthalmologist was greatly concerned that 58% of the injuries he discovered were VISION THREATENING. Study our diagram of the eye. (Figure 11-A)

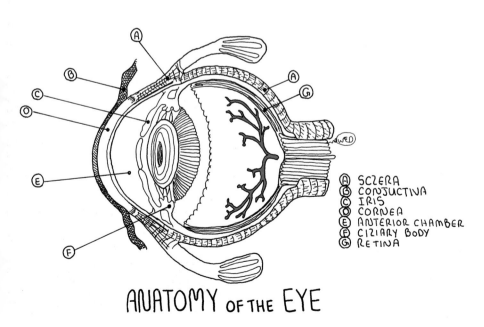

(A) SCLERA
(B) CONJUCTIVA
(C) IRIS
(D) CORNEA
(E) ANTERIOR CHAMBER
(F) CIZIARY BODY
(G) RETINA

ANATOMY OF THE EYE

Figure 11-A: Anatomy of the eye

Many structures in the eye are vulnerable to injury but, importantly, many of the serious, dangerous, vision-threatening injuries may not be immediately evident to the athlete. These are treacherous because they sneak in to steal vision very slowly and dimly—like a "thief in the night." These "slow-stealers" are not necessarily painful, making them all the more dangerous. The skills of a specialist are required to discover defects. You can't trust your intuition on this one! In comparison to a broken nose, finger, or toe—no noticeable evidence may exist. Weakening and collapse of structures like the retina and minor increases of pressure in the eye due to angle recession may cause no pain. Because we possess two eyes and a very adaptable brain—minor defects in vision are subtly compensated for "in house" by our brain without fuses blowing and alarms sounding. (A frog doesn't know he is being cooked if the water is **slowly** heated). Always check one eye at a time for accuracy.

THREE MECHANISMS OF INJURY

Before we go into specifics, I'll explain the three common mechanisms of injury.

1. **Direct contact** (coup)—Coup is direct injury caused by a blow or punch. In wrestling and grappling, contestants are exposed to fast, unplanned movements of the hands and fingers as two bodies move and shift in their efforts to gain advantageous position. An inadvertent poke in the eye is dangerous and painful. Because boxers are gloved, the often offending digit, by default, becomes the thumb. Generally, this category includes **visible** insults to exterior structures such as **eyelids,** abrasions of the **cornea,** and visible blood beneath the conjunctiva. Direct blows that angle inward from a movement such as a hooking punch, can transmit forces to deeper structures. Blood that is visible in the anterior chamber is termed **hyphema.** Hyphema has been linked to **angle recession** which can lead to **glaucoma.**

2. **Contrecoup** causes injury distal from the original contact point and may be understood as a line of force traversing the eye and causing damage at all interfaces. Wave-like contrecoup forces (identical to injury producing circumstances in the brain) are held responsible for injury and scarring of the lens. Such defects are termed **cataracts.** Be warned that

although cataracts are associated most commonly with aging they can exist as a consequence of youthful trauma.

3. **Globe distortion**—Have you ever rolled an orange or tangerine on the kitchen counter to loosen up the skin in an effort to more easily peel it away from the fruit? One has simply compressed and deformed this circular structure in order to release bonds that connect the various layers. A poke or punch to the eye can actually flatten and deform the globe. **Retinal tears** originate as the vision-critical, image collecting retina layer peels off the back of the eye. The plaster is cracked, the paint has peeled, the window shade has rolled up. Vision is lost. Tears and buckles of the retina can vary in size. Earthquakes shake foundations and destabilize layered materials. Punches can produce similar consequences on human anatomy.

Dr. Giovanazzo has clearly documented these mechanisms and resultant defects during his evaluations of professional boxers for the New York State Athletic Commission. 58% of the tested boxers were also stricken with **more than one** category of eye injury.

USA BOXING GUIDELINES

USA Boxing has dutifully listed guidelines for their competitors. Wrestlers and grapplers need not argue concerning their restrictions on eye wear or glasses. Many of us have been absolutely inspired by the courageous (and superbly talented) blind athletes who successfully compete on the mat. Doesn't that confirm the supremely developed sense of touch, reaction, and anticipation that defines the elite wrestler? No argument from them about the need for glasses. USA Boxing bans glasses and few would question this. On the other hand, sparring martial artists can tolerate the wearing of visionware that is appropriately designed with safety in mind. Shatterproof, well padded, secured glasses are available and must be utilized. Boxers blind in one eye are prohibited. The definition of blind is defined as **uncorrected** vision of 20/400. A boxer with **corrected** visual acuity worse than 20/60 in either eye is disqualified. Currently, boxers with uncorrected vision between 20/20 and 20/400 may be permitted to wear soft contact lenses. I do have several problems with this ruling.

1. If a lens becomes dislodged during the heat of a bout, how does a gloved boxer relocate his lens? Is his coach, unfamiliar with contact use, going to poke a dirty finger into the boxer's eye and shove a lens about? How do you sterilize and re-insert a lens that has fallen to the mat? How long a time-out is allowed for everyone to crawl about the mat searching for the dropped "needle in a haystack"? Do the ring girls get drafted for this chore? Will they run their nylons? **(In the pre-bout physical a boxer should be asked if he wears contact lenses. If so, does he have anyone who can replace the lost lens? Did he bring spare lenses? Spare lenses and solutions should be mandatory for the boxers using them.)**

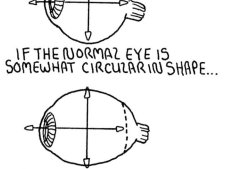

IF THE NORMAL EYE IS SOMEWHAT CIRCULAR IN SHAPE...

THE EYE OF THE NEARSIGHTED PERSON IS MORE OVOID OR ELONGATED IN SHAPE......

Figure 11-B: Normal eye and nearsighted eye

2. If the lens is not replaced, doesn't that boxer compete with a compromised visual acuity?

3. The eyeball that requires glasses is shaped in such a manner as to be at greater risk for injury. If the normal eye is somewhat circular in shape, the eye of a nearsighted person is more oval or elongated in shape (Figure 11-B). This protruding eye is more prominently exposed to the mechanisms of injury that we detailed just paragraphs ago.

Amateur boxers with a history of retinal detachment or cataract formation (surgically corrected or not) shall not box. Martial artists and law enforcement trainees should take all precautions necessary to protect their vision. Know your eyeglass options!

INJURY CARE

It is reported that 100,000 eye injuries each year are sports related, i.e., all sports, not just combat sports. Most eye injuries originate from basketball, baseball, swimming, and racket sports.

ABRASIONS OF THE CORNEA—"SCRATCHED EYE"

The injured cells of the cornea produce pain, sensitivity to bright light, and tearing. The scratched cornea is roughened and radiates pain each time one blinks. Many victims swear that a foreign object has gotten in their eye (dust, gravel, rocks, mountains)! The more they rub, scratch, open, close, wash, and fuss, the worse the scratched surface becomes as it rubs against the inner eyelid. The history of injury is important. Was it wind-blown dust or a poke/rub across the eye? A fluorescein dye that demonstrates a green stain on the injured cells confirms the diagnosis of a scratch. Initially, use large volumes of water to thoroughly irrigate out any foreign materials. Once the appropriate diagnosis is confirmed by a doctor, treatment consists of a topical antibiotic ointment and a cotton eye pressure patch. Corneal cells heal very rapidly and great progress is made overnight. A patched eye doesn't blink often and the eye is allowed to settle down. Don't put topical anesthetic eye drops in your eye once the diagnosis has been assured and treatment started. If your eye is numb, the natural reaction to pain is lost and unrealized movements could promote severe damage. **Minor contact lens** related corneal abrasions may not need to be patched according to one expert. **The offending contact lens should be removed for healing to occur.**

CONJUNCTIVAL HEMORRHAGE

A superficial collection of blood in the white part of the eye usually resolves in 1½ to 2 weeks. These are benign and don't require treatment. (Figure 11-C)

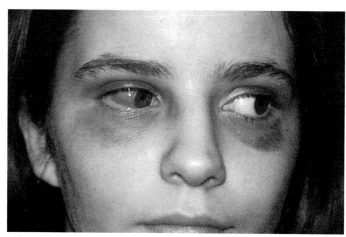

Figure 11-C: Conjunctival hemorrhage

CONJUNCTIVITIS

Conjunctivitis is infection of the conjunctiva which causes redness and pus production. Sometimes this is called "pink eye." Don't compete with other athletes. The infections, bacterial or viral, are very contagious and might endanger the entire team.

TRAUMATIC IRITIS

Blunt trauma to the eye can injure the colored iris or ciliary body. Symptoms are tearing, pain, and light sensitivity. The pupil of the injured eye may remain dilated and not contract when exposed to light. Eye specialists must be consulted.

HYPHEMA

Blunt injury can cause blood to collect in the anterior chamber. Other equally dangerous injuries often accompany this finding. A doctor must be consulted. Usually bed rest, elevation of the head of the bed, and medicines are utilized. Re-bleeding will occur if the athlete doesn't heed the doctor's orders. The critical time for a re-bleed is the first 72 hours after injury.

FOREIGN BODIES

Dust or dirt in an eye is quite an unpleasant experience. This object can scratch the cornea. Further rubbing of the eye adds "injury to the insult" rather than "insult to injury." Thorough irrigation with water or saline should suffice if one also lifts the lid to allow trapped particles to be rinsed away. Sometimes a doctor will gently swab the area with a moistened cotton swab. Metal splinters require a surgeon to remove them under local anesthesia and magnification.

RETINAL TEARS

A torn retina should be considered a possibility should an athlete report flashes of light or sensation of a curtain being pulled down over his/her eye. Timely examination by an expert will detect a loss of sight in a portion of the usual visual field and hopefully avert any further or permanent vision loss. Doctors must use medicines to fully dilate your pupil in order to visualize the early peripheral retinal tears present in boxers.

PTOSIS

David approached me at my ringside seat following his win in the Olympic Trials. "Check out my eye, Doc" was his request.

A drooping, lazy eyelid was apparent and subsequent, detailed exams revealed no problem with his eye or vision. (Figure 11-D) This boxer was enthusiastic having won the Olympic Trials and an enviable elite spot on the USA Olympic Team. Several blows to his eye the day prior

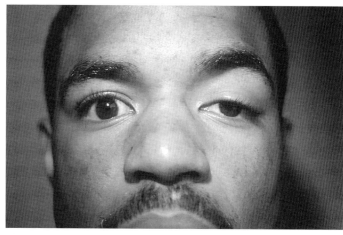

Figure 11-D: Olympic Champion, David Reid with ptosis (drooping eyelid)

caused his eyelid to partially droop, but it totally corrected as he slept. Despite winning the finals, a few shots landed recreating the deformity. Although his true vision was unimpaired, his exposure to right hooks was risky. A partial curtain was covering punches traveling high and to his left. In order to compensate, he instinctively elevated his chin in order to enhance his field of view—a no-no in boxing. The chin must be safely tucked in to avoid devastating knock-out punches. David was so skilled and fast of reflex that he effectively controlled the situation.

Follow-up exams by elite referrals confirm a partial tear in the levator muscle, a small muscle unit that elevates the lid. This condition is the best of all scenarios and can heal on its own. If spontaneous recovery fails to occur, a somewhat minor reattachment surgery remains an option.

The differential diagnosis includes Horner's syndrome, brain injury, and third nerve palsy. David is fortunate and became the 1996 Olympic gold medal winner of the light-middleweight category. *USA Today* refers to him as "the 156-pounder with a droopy left eyelid."

HOW TO ASSESS TROUBLE

1. **TEST YOUR VISION**—Try reading a newspaper to test **close vision.** Test one eye at a time! Try reading **distant** objects. Test one eye at a time.

2. **PUPIL TESTING**—Does your pupil **contract** when a bright light shines in each eye? Does it expand in the dark? In **similar** light intensi-

ties, are your pupil **sizes equal** left-to-right? Is your pupil highly sensitive to bright light? This indicates problems.

3. **CORNEA CHECK**—Is blood present in the anterior chamber, just under the cornea **(hyphema)**? Are foreign **objects imbedded** in the cornea? Under magnification imbedded metal splinters, even after removal, may leave a permanently discolored **"rust ring."** Out of interest, boxers who are slow to return to their former performance levels after a layoff are said to have "ring rust."

4. **CONJUNCTIVA SURVEY**—Is there **blood** under the clear conjunctiva that discreetly overlies the white sclera (conjunctival hemorrhage)? Is pus present indicating infection? Are **foreign bodies** present under your upper or lower eyelid causing **reddish** irritation of your conjunctiva?

5. **MOVE IT**—Look upward, downward, and towards each side. Do both eyes travel in a coordinated rhythm? If they don't, your clue is **double vision.** Fractures of the orbital floor can entrap the overlying muscles. The most common reason for an orbital floor fracture remains a direct blow to the upper cheek.

6. **PAIN**—Your body is trying to tell you something. Are you listening?

7. Persistent **WATERING** of the eye.

GO TO THE DOCTOR (OPHTHALMOLOGIST), AS SUGGESTED BY JAY C. ERIE, M.D., IN *THE PHYSICIAN & SPORTSMEDICINE JOURNAL,* IF:
- A foreign body cannot be washed out
- A layer of blood is seen in the anterior chamber
- Impaired near or far vision
- A pupil that is irregular, non-circular or sluggishly reactive as compared to the opposite side
- Double vision
- Cuts on the lids
- Shattered glasses or contact lens tears
- Any problem perceived as vision threatening
- Unremittent pain

Chapter 12

Infectious Diseases

HERPES SIMPLEX

I hate to do it, but that's my job! I recently disallowed the "main event" participant of an "anything goes" martial arts tournament. The promoters were not happy but accepted my explanation as respectfully as the athlete. I don't take pride in halting a competitor. I thoroughly enjoy watching a skilled performance! Several weeks ago I was forced to "D.Q." (disqualify) an otherwise healthy, well-trained, and confident young man from participating in a national boxing championship tournament for his age group.

Why did I stop these athletes? During pre-bout physicals I noticed freshly-formed and oozing blisters about the lips and cheek area. Both were otherwise in superb shape and had trained intensively to become fit, fast, and lean. In addition, effort was expended by the boxer to make weight for the 7:00 A.M. weigh-ins which were scheduled in conjunction with the physical exams. This was no small contest. Winning on three consecutive days—quarter-finals, semi-finals, and a championship round—would position him as #1 in his age bracket for USA Boxing. Lots of pressure on this teenager! He failed to recall ever having this condition in the past. This outbreak of "cold sores," "fever blisters," was his initial episode.

Herpes Simplex is a common condition with approximately 90% of American adults by age 50 testing positive for antibodies. Usually this virus presents as the common "cold sore" agonizingly conspicuous near the margin of the lips. (Figure 12-A) Most individuals will experience one or two attacks per year with each attack lasting five to fourteen days. Most usually, the initial fluid-filled, angry, oozing blisters will crust over and fade away, leaving no scars or evidence of this deeply established virus.

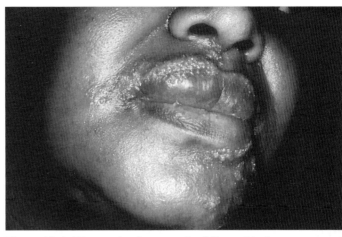

Figure 12-A: Herpes simplex — active blistered lesions can spread the virus

This is a **permanent condition.** Between attacks the virus hides inactively in nerve endings called dorsal root nerve ganglia and sleeps a dormant slumber. It hibernates within its permanent den. When the individual experiences stress and the body's natural immunity is weakened, the sleeping bear retraces its steps up to the skin and growls for five to fourteen days. Stresses commonly include exposure to sunlight (U-V rays), physical challenges, weight loss, and emotional pressure. Doesn't this mirror many of the training challenges imposed upon a competitive athlete? Usually one can sense a premonition of outbreak several days before the skin manifestations. This preliminary tingling, burning discomfort on the skin will be recognized by a patient familiar with the situation. The lesions will be clustered as grouped vesicles (bubbly blisters) surrounded by redness and crusting. Scab formation represents the final inactive stage.

So you now ask—why is this serious enough to force a boxing, wrestling, or martial arts competitor out of a major tournament? Many reasons. First of all, this is a permanent, life-time, affliction caused by Herpes Simplex, Type I. Herpes Simplex, Type II, is a Herpes virus responsible for genital herpes—the cause of tormenting blistering on the penis or female genitalia. Recently, due to current sexual habits, types I and II are so interchangeable that few useful reasons remain to sub-classify them. The virus is shed and highly transmissible during the contagious stages of blistering and oozing. Any skin-to-

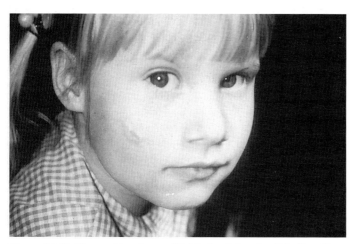

Figure 12-B: Herpes Simplex — "A Mother's Loving Kiss" — How active herpes can be spread

skin contact can spread this permanent virus elsewhere to other skin sites on the host's or opponent's body. This affliction isn't isolated to the mouth or lips. Some doctors carry the dormant virus on their fingertip because they dutifully examined an infected patient before the days of knowledgeable sterile technique. A sad photograph shows a child's cheek, angrily infected where mom "planted" an otherwise loving kiss. (Figure 12-B)

Grapplers and wrestlers are classically recognized as high risk for their extreme skin-to-skin abrasive contact. In fact, recognized outbreaks of lesions on the forehead, chin, neck, or shoulders have been labeled HERPES GLADIATORUM, a skin disease of these modern gladiators. A rather well-known mass outbreak occurred during a wrestling camp in 1989. Of the 60 infected wrestlers, the lesions were distributed as follows:

- Head—44 athletes
- Extremities—25 athletes
- Trunk—17 athletes
- Eye—5 athletes

In a separate survey of 2,625 college wrestlers, 7.6% developed active herpes simplex during a single wrestling season in 1985.

What else can happen? The motivating realization that blindness can result from corneal involvement caused me to encourage USA Boxing to list "active herpes lesions" as a disqualifying condition in their 1994 Official Rulebook. The membership was highly cooperative in accepting our committee's recommendation and few coaches complained. If this virus spreads to the eye, the lesions may cloudily scar the cornea resulting in a loss of vision. Advice similar to choosing an intimate partner exists—know your "wrestling" partner. Whether in training or competition, observe for obvious skin lesions especially on the face. These can't be hidden!

When I was actively competing in body-building in the early 1980's, one of my fellow competitors and occasional workout buddies began having some knee problems. In the mid-eighties, having known me and feeling confident that I would give him "extra special care," he requested a knee exam. Subsequent visits, a failure of improvement, and scans suggested a torn meniscus ("cartilage"). Arthroscopic surgery was performed by me, and I felt quite pleased and confident that his problem had been positively addressed and he could now regain full athletic activity. I felt very rewarded to have helped a buddy achieve a healthy return to an activity he loved. He represented one of the emotional fulfillments that guided me into medicine and through the many arduous years of medical and surgical training. After all, I had in essence, traded all of my 20's (third decade) for the future rewards that medicine promised.

Four or five days after the outpatient surgery, his frantic and tearful young wife phoned my office from the intensive care waiting room. Larry was lying unresponsive in a coma within the neuro-intensive care unit. I rushed to evaluate him and sort out his sudden change in status. Larry was comatose, intubated, and unable to provide any hints. Larry's wife could only provide relevant information that he began feeling dizzy about two days ago and that he drifted into a deep slumber and fever the morning of admission. You can imagine that my first action was removal of my surgical dressing and checking of his knee for infection or a treatable complication. Removal of his sterile dressing and compression wrap revealed a knee that was remarkably well healed, not even showing the expected swelling that accompanies surgery. His knee was thankfully benign and completely safe. I could provide little additional assistance as his care was now in the hands of the neurologist. My surgery utilized standard general anesthesia with no invasive spinal procedures. Subsequent tests were negative, except for a spinal tap that eventually confirmed a **herpes** encephalitis (brain infection) with no known cause. He died. Somehow the herpes virus had invaded his spinal cord system. I don't know his past history of genital and/or skin involvement. His is an extremely rare but sad case. Don't jump to the conclusion that oral herpes is a fatal disease. Herpes cold sores are very common, just avoid spreading this permanent virus to unknowing competitors. When a coach or athlete argues against disqualification because of "a stupid fever blister," I share with them my rationalization for the decision but silence my deeper personal sadness and questions of "why him?" A doctor must suppress emotional scars of horrible personal tragedies witnessed year by year, so that he may continue functioning in a scientific and rational fashion. Athletes, in turn, must suppress human frailties in their quest to challenge their multiple moving parts with machine-like demands.

Some good news exists. Once the lesions are well scabbed-over and dry, although visible, the chance of transmission has disappeared and one may safely compete. Clinically we use a cotton swab to rub across the lesion. If blisters, fluid, or soft breakable scabs are present—no competition is allowed. If rubbing demonstrates a solid, well adhering, dry scab, then full activity is safe. Additionally, a new anti-virus drug, ACYCLOVIR, if taken in the several hour window **BEFORE** the skin blisters appear, shortens the course of the outbreak approximately 50%. The usual dose is 200mg orally 5 times daily for 5 days. See your doctor for specifics. Hence, if one alertly senses the itching, tingling, burning and utilizes this medicine, it is possible to decrease the total length of contagious state and heal by a deadline for competition. It is advised that an athlete keep the medicine on hand to prevent a delay in administration. On rare occasions, preventative use of the medicine prior to a stressful major competition or elite tournament situation is an option. Seek information from your family doctor.

IMPETIGO

Impetigo is a **bacterial** superficial skin infection caused by the common germs staph (staphylococcus) and strep (streptococcus). If recognized at a reasonable time, local wound care and common antibiotics are effective. Any outbreak of impetigo among a high school wrestling team can wipe out and ground the entire team. This is highly contagious and identified as blisters with yellow pus that dries into a honey-colored crust. Sorry for being so colorful and graphic. (Figure 12-C) Its prevention is rather basic and easy. Proper hygiene is mandatory. Cleanse wrestling or grappling mats and equipment like headgear, gloves, and uniforms daily with antiseptic solutions. One accountable person must be responsible for these duties. Personal hygiene and non-stinky clothes will decrease any likelihood of transmission. Participants with suspicious skin lesions should be eliminated from contact activities. Minor unhealed lesions do not necessarily condemn an athlete to total exclu-

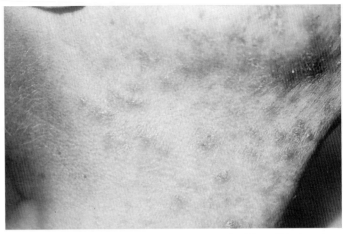

Figure 12-C: Impetigo — easily treated with antibiotics

sion. If the affected area is well covered, the combat athlete can still maintain fitness activities like jogging, jump rope, weight training, or stationary bicycle work-outs. Seek early care and professional advice to minimize confusion in identifying herpes, impetigo, and other disorders at their various stages. Coaches have the responsibility to screen their own athletes to prevent outbreaks among uninformed competitors.

H.I.V. AND AIDS (Figure 12-D)

There is so much to say and so little time to say it! Becoming H.I.V. positive (infected) indicates that an individual has suffered exposure to the Human Immunodeficiency Virus. Initial symptoms may only manifest as the "flu." After this episode, an individual may appear absolutely healthy; failing to exhibit any signs or symptoms of illness for a duration of ten years. An H.I.V. infected individual

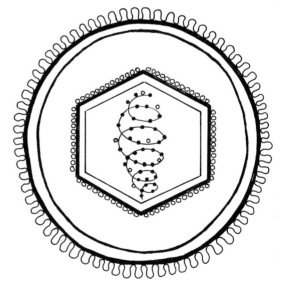

Figure 12-D: Representation of HIV virus

can transmit this eventually fatal disease for ten years and yet remain fully competitive and healthy-appearing. A deceptive existence fashions and fabricates the very frightening and challenging "mask" of this disease.

The most infectious periods exist during the initial 30 days after exposure (undiagnosed) and late in the disease when actual symptoms appear. A carrier has been estimated to be 100 to 1,000 times more infectious during these time periods. Only when the victim's internal defenses crumble to the continuous growth and onslaught of this constantly replicating virus does the term—AIDS (Acquired Immune Deficiency Syndrome) apply. Symptoms are now blatantly visible.

We, as a society, misguided by our trusted "advisors" have discarded our "golden opportunity" to contain it. Selfish, "minority rights" activists have pressured the American Medical Association into breaking their age-old public health rules scientifically established to limit the spread of disease. The time-honored principles that effectively controlled tuberculosis, typhus, and syphilis among an innocent populous, have been unwisely and fatally discarded to show preferential treatment to a tiny minority. The right to health among 99% of our population has been subordinated to the vocal biases of a minute minority.

In a few short years, several hundred non-isolated, irresponsible carriers spread a preventable virus that now (1995) infects 1 in 80 American males between the ages of 18 and 35. One in 600 women within this same age bracket serves as a carrier. They are the most rapidly enlarging subgroup due to heterosexual spread. After attending my lecture to elite boxing coaches about the H.I.V. outbreak, a coach (name and location withheld) returned to his gym and obtained the funding to blood test his athletes. Several months later he reported to me that two of his active boxers were confirmed to test positive. My words were not wasted! The risk of transmission from male to female is almost twice as great as from woman to man. While in France serving as ringside physician for our U.S. Team, my French physician counterpart estimated a similar infection rate among French males.

Thankfully, there has never been a scientifically documented case of H.I.V. transmission during athletic competition (as of 1996). A rumored transmission between two Italian soccer players has failed to support, and undeniably confirm, initial suspicions. The two players did collide with resultant head-to-head lacerations that profusely bled. However, no confirmed cases are documented in the world's medical literature. Thankfully, H.I.V. is extremely difficult to transmit in a casual setting, which includes athletic competition. Because the virus is so fragile, it does not survive when exposed to air for any period of time. *NO* cases have ever been confirmed by sporting events. Think LIFESTYLE, not sport!

Let's maintain a non-hysterical scientific perspective! The undeniable modes of transmission are:

1. Homosexual activity

2. Unprotected heterosexual activity

3. Drug abuse and shared needles

4. Hospital workers either inadvertently stuck with contaminated needles or directly splashed into mouth or eye by contaminated sources

5. Contaminated blood transfusion or blood products

6. Contaminated organ recipients

At this point in time, about thirty-five health care workers have sero-converted (tested positive for H.I.V.) after a "splash." That is, they were not stuck, but contaminated fluids were splashed upon or into at-risk mucous membranes—eyes, nose, mouth, and non-intact skin. Repeat! Don't panic as athletes! It has been estimated that an NFL football player would need to play in over one million (1,000,000) games to be "at risk." Although the transmission risk in athletic competition is infinitesimal, the risk is not 0%. Therefore, prudent universal precautions are highly advised. If athletic risk can be estimated, the combat sports rank among the highest for possible transmission scenario! USA Boxing has ruled that a referee **MAY** (not must) stop a bout where two boxers are actively bleeding or one boxer is bleeding and his opponent has open cuts or abrasions. USA Wrestling allows injury time-outs of five minutes to control bleeding. Grossly bloody uniforms should be changed. Bloody clothing can be washed with household detergents in a conventional manner. USA Wrestling does not allow athletes and health care attendants known to be infected with H.I.V. to compete or administer to bleeding athletes. USA Boxing also excludes H.I.V. athletes from competition.

Bloody wounds should be cleansed with an antiseptic and the wound sterilely covered. Gross blood spills onto mats and equipment should be cleansed with soapy water followed by a CLOROX solution diluted 1:10 with water. Daily equipment and mats should be cleaned with this fresh 1:10 mixture of CLOROX and water. (One part CLOROX in ten parts WATER). Soap and alcohol **DO NOT** kill the AIDS virus. Note that the CLOROX/WATER solution must be re-mixed daily as it deactivates each 24 hours. Clearly label each bottle of solution so that it is not mistaken for drinkable fluids. Spittoons should contain killing solutions (Clorox) because of the expected blood-tinged spit.

Gloves should be worn by coaches, trainers, and referees when contacting:

    1. Blood

    2. Blood-tinged products

    3. Open wounds

    4. Mucous membranes

    5. Cleaning of spills

Essentially, only blood and sexual secretions, have been documented to carry the AIDS virus. Those body fluids that have **not** been implicated in infection transmission are:

    1. Sweat

    2. Tears

    3. Vomitus

    4. Sputum

    5. Urine

    6. Saliva—recent evidence as virus containing

At this time, no universal precautions are recommended if exposed to these body fluids. It is most appropriate that blood, bloody sponges, and grossly contaminated clothing be discarded in red, labeled, biohazard bags.

Several concluding points must be emphasized:

1. The behavior of athletes in off-the-field activities is dramatically and infinitely more critical to H.I.V. exposure risk than on-field sports.

2. Required testing is complex and problematic. There is never a guarantee of a non-carrier state. It takes about three weeks to six months for currently utilized blood tests to turn positive after an exposure. A negative test today doesn't guarantee that an individual wasn't exposed the pre-

ceding night. Therefore, universal precautions are always indicated for safety. It is thought that the greatest chance of spreading the infection occurs during the first month of exposure and years later during the frank illness stage. But risk remains overwhelming at any time during those "silent" years.

3. The inherent injury dangers of the combat arts far outweigh the infinitesimal risks of H.I.V. exposure.

OUR NEXT BOUT
BY: JOSEPH J. ESTWANIK, M.D. © 1993

He is deceptively small but powerful
A newcomer, but we do have recent footage of his bouts:
    he trains in a very unconventional manner
Relentless, with an ever-improving record
A very adaptable opponent, recent changes in his
    techniques are reported.
His trainers are rumored to be naive, selfish, and
    uncaring
His ring attire can vary from bland to flashy
He will lull you into underestimation because of very
    subtle moves
You will be tempted into letting down your guard as he
    "hits below the belt"
He becomes ferocious at the first sight of blood
He has a jaw of granite—we don't have a punch that
    will take him out
Our game plan: The best offense is a good defense;
    expect a 20-Rounder!

… A.I.D.S.

HEPATITIS

In contrast to the very rare chance of contracting H.I.V. during sport (rated as infinitestimal—i.e. chances so low that they are nearly incalculable), hepatitis is a disease of realistic concern. Hepatitis indicates that a virus has attacked and damaged the liver. There are many types or forms of hepatitis but types A, B, and C are most common.

HEPATITIS A

Hepatitis A (H.A.V.) is the "contaminated" food and water form. The incubation is two to six weeks and spread through the fecal-oral route.

HEPATITIS B

Hepatitis B (H.B.V.) follows the recognized transmission routes to which we have been sensitized because of AIDS. It is calculated that H.B.V. is many times more infectious than AIDS. H.B.V. is more concentrated in blood than is H.I.V. A single c.c. of blood infected with H.B.V. may contain 100 million infectious doses of virus, whereas H.I.V. infested blood contains only 100— several 1000 particles/c.c. The time of incubation is one to six months and flu-like pre-symptoms last two to six weeks. Symptoms include dark urine, light stools, and liver tenderness. Long term complications can cause the infected individual to enter a chronic carrier state in 6% to 10% of cases. This means that despite an individual appearing recovered and healthy—he can continue to shed the virus and infect others. The long term health conditions can result in CIRRHOSIS (a scarred, damaged, poorly functioning liver in 15% to 30% of cases) or the terminal situation of liver cancer. Feared transmission pathways include infection by receiving a blood transfusion, sexual contact, saliva, and such apparently harmless routes as sharing a shaving razor or a toothbrush.

There is good news! A vaccine exists to protect us from this potentially fatal disease. As a surgeon I quickly jumped at the chance to become immunized. Sadly, many dedicated physicians and surgeons have contracted this virus while treating patients. Surgeons are at great risk from inadvertent needle sticks during surgery. On many occasions I have been stuck despite my constant awareness of safety technique. I'm afraid this is a part of the game for a busy surgeon. Surgeons have died from any one of their unexpected sticks.

It is now recommended that children receive Hepatitis B doses in conjunction with their required "childhood" immunizations. Many school systems are now providing, in cooperation with County Health Departments, Hepatitis B immunizations to children once attaining a specified grade level. For example, the State of North Carolina is providing the Hepatitis B series to all sixth graders (11 and 12 year olds) who wish to receive the injections. This will continue until the year 2004 in the hopes that at sexual maturation all children will have been immunized against this fatal disease.

All at-risk groups—including athletes, coaches, trainers—must be immunized. The vaccine is a three part series. The doses are given by injection at 0 - 1- 6 months. Miss any one of these three and the vaccine may not "take." Don't miss or skip a dose. I've definitely completed my full series! Use the same safety considerations for H.B.V. that have been dramatically publicized by the press for H.I.V.

HEPATITIS C

Hepatitis C (H.C.V.) has an incubation of two to six weeks and represents 20% to 40% of acute viral hepatitis in the U.S.A. 60% of people infected have no known or remembered history of exposure, although high risk groups include:

1. an exposure to blood

2. a household (sharing a toothbrush or razor) or sexual exposure to persons with hepatitis.

HUMAN BITE

"You are better to be bitten by a dog than a human" is a quote that startled me as an intern during my emergency room rotation. But, how true!

A fist or finger cut by a tooth may appear as a "nothing" but can progress into a serious situation. In my experience, serving as a physician for the ULTIMATE FIGHTING CHAMPIONSHIPS, I learned of just such a complication from an earlier series of bouts. Despite the more blatant concerns of serious injury when "Reality" fighting exploded into action, a former participant with a "tooth" cut on his hand became the only hospitalized casualty. He required I.V. antibiotics and could have progressed into an open surgical drainage. A multitude of exotic germs populate the mouth. All prosper in such a warm and moist environment. Isn't it a miracle we have all survived kissing? I guess we must pick our poison.

A benign appearing cut on the knuckle must be thoroughly cleansed. Most emergency rooms choose **NOT** to suture closed a cut from this saliva contaminated source. If the cut is left purposely open and infection does occur, drainage can escape and not be forced deeper into the tissues by pressure. Pus must be allowed to escape. Pus under pressure is destructive and dangerous. Definitely visit your doctor early if you suspect infection by such a source.

EXERCISE DURING AN ILLNESS

(This material is adapted by Dr. W. A. Primos from "Sports and Exercise During Acute Illness," *Phys. SportsMed,* 1996: 24[1]: 44-52, by permission of McGraw-Hill, Inc.)

It is well known that regular exercise can improve health, but even elite athletes are grounded by sicknesses like the flu, measles, and colds. Usually during an illness, one does not feel like exercising. However some athletes, especially those who are competitively motivated, have reasons to continue training or competing during an illness. They feel that they will fall out of shape if they skip a few days in the gym. Athletes may have an important game or competition that they fear missing. What is the best avenue to follow during an illness? Should you rest or is it o.k. to exercise? Can it be dangerous to exercise with an illness? Are there specific types of diseases that are especially hazardous for exercisers?

Research studies have shown that exercise causes worsening of respiratory illnesses like the common cold, bronchitis, and pneumonia. Intense exercise during such a sickness can cause increased cough, wheezing, and shortness of breath.

People who have illnesses with fever, vomiting, and/or diarrhea may get dehydrated during their illness. Intense exercise causes additional loss of fluid through sweating. Heat builds up because the body can't cool itself down properly. This sets one up for heatstroke which can be lethal. Due to the risk of heatstroke, intense exercise should be avoided by anyone with an illness that consists of diarrhea, vomiting, or fever. If you are running a fever, it is not wise to workout. Rest, use acetaminophen, ibuprofen, or aspirin, and drink fluids to maximize your recovery. Children should not ingest aspirin during febrile illnesses to avoid the rare disease of Reye's Syndrome. Viral illnesses with the classic sore throat, runny nose, and sinus congestion are not improved by antibiotics. Should unusual manifestations appear, obviously schedule a visit with your doctor.

Sometimes a virus, called coxsackievirus, can cause an illness that mimics the flu. This virus may infect the heart muscles and cause myocarditis. If people with this heart infection participate in strenuous activities, they may suffer heart failure or a heart attack which can kill them. Due to this possible complication, it is recommended that individuals suffering flu-like illness with fever and muscle aches avoid strenuous exercise until they feel well.

Another fairly common disease that may have a severe complication is infectious mononucleosis or "mono." Fatigue, prolonged sore throat, and swollen lymph nodes could announce mono (mononucleosis). An enlarged spleen, which often accompanies this illness, is a definite indication to avoid contact activities as a ruptured spleen causes potentially fatal internal bleeding. This swollen, spongy spleen may rupture or "pop" during strenuous athletics, especially contact sports where the abdomen may be hit forcefully. Therefore, athletes should avoid strenuous and contact sports for at least one month after coming down with mono, assuming their spleen is not found enlarged by their examining doctor. A common blood test can easily screen for mono infections.

A good general guideline for determining whether or not it is safe to participate in physical activities during your illness has been developed. It is called the "neck check" (Eichner 1). If all of your symptoms are **ABOVE** the neck, (Figure 12-E) like runny nose, scratchy throat, or an earache, then exercise is probably safe. Start exercising at low intensity for several minutes. If you don't begin to feel worse, then increase the exertion level. However, if symptoms are located **BELOW** the neck, (Figure 12-E) such as muscle aches, fever, chills, weakness, diarrhea, or a deep cough, avoid exercise. By resting you can avoid worsening your illness and suffering severe complications. You will also recover faster with rest because you are giving your body a chance to heal itself rather than direct its energy for exercise.

Another factor that you should consider, if you harbor an illness, is whether

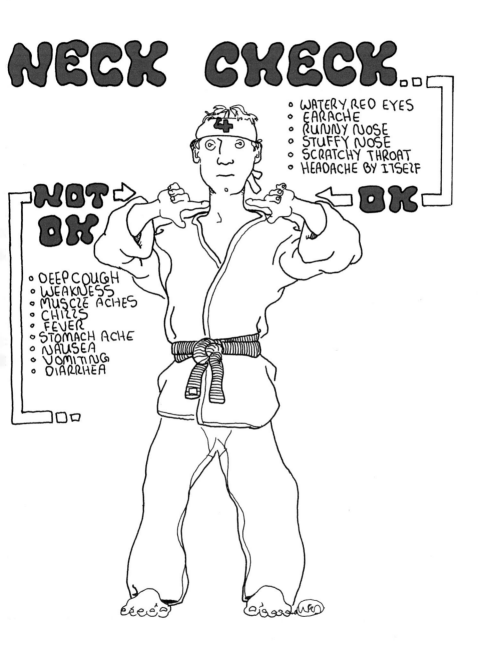

Figure 12-E: "Neck Check" — symptoms above neck / symptoms below neck

or not you may selfishly infect other participants on your team or in your gym. Some illnesses can be easily transferred to others through invisible respiratory droplets. Measles and common colds are such diseases. These viruses can be transmitted through the air when the infected person coughs or sneezes near someone else. Therefore, people with measles should not be around others until four days after the rash first appears.

There are many innocent ways in which illnesses are unknowingly spread to others such as by shared ice buckets, drinking containers, and towels. Infections can be effectively decreased by the use of disposable cups, individual water bottles, and towels.

[1]. Eichner, ER: "Infection, immunity, and exercise," *Phys. SportsMed* 1993: 21 (1): 125 -135.

Chapter 13

Spine

What a topic to explain! It has been estimated that an extremely large percentage of Americans will have low back pain on some occasion during their lifetime. Let's not incriminate athletics as the bad guy. Housework, occupational demands, driving, and even a **lack of exercise** can be included as causative factors. So, should you be saddled with this malady, a well supervised tune-up program in aerobics or aerobic boxing (Box-ergenics™) can still put you on the right track.

VERTEBRAE ANATOMY

First, the chassis set-up. (Figure 13-A) Vertebrae are the bony building blocks, the frame, that hold us in an upright position. Unless you actually sustain a severe injury that fractures the spine, the bones themselves will rarely cause a problem. Unless osteoporosis or a lack of exercise creates premature stress fractures, healthy vertebrae can be expected to happily support our frame into a perky old age.

Osteoporosis is abnormal thinning of the bones due to a low level of calcium within the microscopic bone tissue. Post-menopausal women are most aggressively affected. The end stage of this "disease includes a decrease in stature (shortening), humped back, rounded shoulders, painful compression fractures within the vertebra and fractures of the arms and legs, often occurring at the wrist and hip. An equally treacherous condition may exist in young, over-exercising, diet-conscious ladies (rarely men). In full pathology, the "female athlete triad" includes osteoporosis, absence or suppression of men-

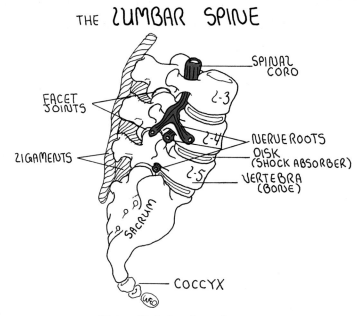

THE LUMBAR SPINE

SPINAL CORD

FACET JOINTS

L-3

ZIGAMENTS

L-4

NERVE ROOTS

DISK (SHOCK ABSORBER)

L-5

VERTEBRA (BONE)

SACRUM

COCCYX

Figure 13-A: Lumbar spine

struation, and eating disorders such as anorexia nervosa, bulimia, and purging. The woman who is a compulsive exerciser, strict dieter (to the point of bulimia and purging), and perpetually envisioning herself as "too fat" risks a lifelong curse of osteoporosis so severe that she will never ever be able to saturate her skeleton with its normal density of minerals (calcium and phosphorous).

We all need a baseline level of body fat to assure the building blocks for health. However, a safe minimum percentage body fat is 7% for youthful wrestlers. A calculated and documented level for elite women swimmers ranged from 14% - 26%. My associate, William A. Primos, Jr., M.D., a member of the American Medical Society for SportsMedicine has pin-pointed the weight loss problem to its bare-bones concern. "It is the starvation and dehydration of the body on the road to pathologic 'low fat' that really hurts you, not THE ARRIVAL AT a specific numerical value for % body fat." Some very healthy athletes (in every sense of the word) carry around an amazingly low amount of body fat. There is no notable research to confirm that a low number dictates bad health in a high performance athlete like Herschel Walker, the pro football player from the University of Georgia. The lesson to be learned is that low absolute numbers aren't exactly synonymous with disease.

The pathologic, ill-advised methods to **arrive** at extreme leanness are what can become distorted, absurd, pathologic, and faulty. Again, use the "mirror test" if you can be trusted to be honest with yourself. Those truly (and possibly fatally ill) with anorexia nervosa (or extreme obesity) have a highly distorted and perverse self image—even when standing stark naked in a full length mirror. With the exception of pathologic over-exercising and under-eating syndromes, a proper exercise program will prevent the gradual leaking of calcium from the bones as women and men approach middle age. One might even visualize that exercise drives circulating calcium into the bones rather than floating unused in the blood stream. That old adage—"use it or lose it"—works again.

DISCS

Our spine's shock absorbers—the discs—are responsible for most of the structural weaknesses within the neck, thoracic spine, and low back. Pain can emanate from (1) the disc, (2) the small paired joints (called the facet joints), and (3) ligaments.

As a youth, your discs are supple, fully inflated shock absorbers filled with a jelly-like center. Imagine a fresh jelly doughnut. As we age our disc by injury or poor posture, the liquid center begins to dry out and travel towards the edge of the doughnut. This asymmetric bulging stretches the disc causing pain and a less efficient absorber for running, sitting, and standing stresses. Imagine traveling down some bumpy unpaved road on tires or shocks that are going flat. The entire chassis shakes, rattles, and creaks. The passengers aren't happy! As the jelly doughnut collapses down and the jelly pokes further outward, nearby structures,

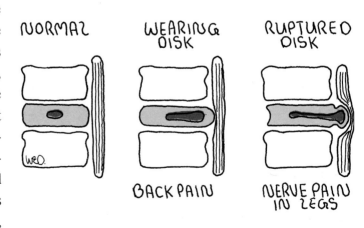

Figure 13-B-1: Ruptured disc

like nerves, can get pressured and squeezed. Now the pain is not only localized to the spine, but shooting down the leg (a condition called sciatica) where the nerve transmits it messages. Suddenly, we have progressed from a "slipped disc" to a "pinched nerve." Nerves are very sensitive to pressure and will quit working which causes a numb foot or weak calf muscles. (Figure 13-B-1 and Figure 13-B-2)

Some individuals are born with durable materials in the spine (40,000 mile rubber on their tires) and will tolerate great forces. Others unfortunately inherit a lower grade of rubber on their tires or thinner formica on their cabinet tops. The less fortunate will develop chronic low back pain and need to modify their workout stresses

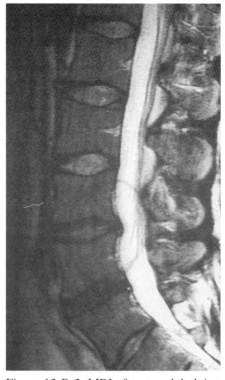

Figure 13-B-2: MRI of ruptured, bulging disc compressing the thecal sac (nerves)

and techniques. Most abdominal work in the Boxergenics™ system is performed with the knees bent, and slow partial sit-up movements to protect the spine. To over-emphasize a point—a single sit-up held for a count of fifty can be just as challenging as 50 individual sit-ups. A single chin-up performed to last 15 seconds may rival 15 single chin-ups. I recommend controlled, slow-movement, bent-knee abdominal exercises. By bending your knees, you relax the iliopsoas muscle which travels from the hips up to the pelvis where it attaches onto the low back (lumbar) vertebrae. Every rapid-fire sit-up performed with the knees straight (like the old Army exercises) directly pulls upon the spine with each repetition. In this negative situation, the hip flexors are yanking on the spinal segments and by-passing the all important abdominal muscles which are actually supportive and protective muscles for the spine. (Figure 13-C) There is no need to perform twisty-turny exercises that rotate far to the left and far to the right. These only accelerate wear on the discs

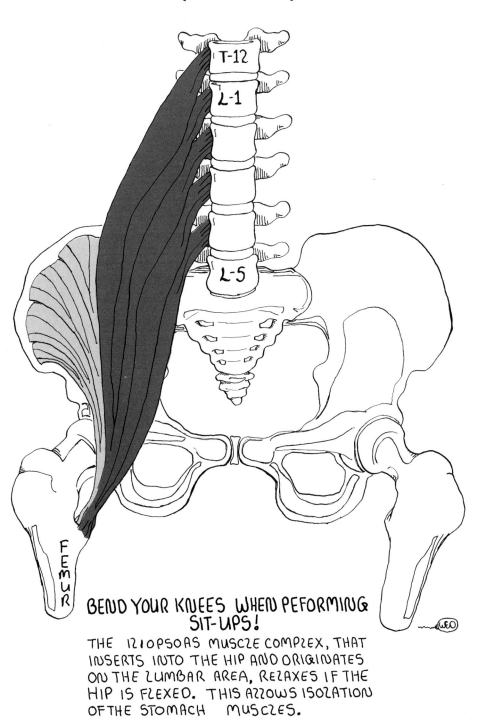

BEND YOUR KNEES WHEN PEFORMING SIT-UPS!
THE ILIOPSOAS MUSCLE COMPLEX, THAT INSERTS INTO THE HIP AND ORIGINATES ON THE LUMBAR AREA, RELAXES IF THE HIP IS FLEXED. THIS ALLOWS ISOLATION OF THE STOMACH MUSCLES.

Figure 13-C: Iliopsoas Muscle Complex — "Bend your knees when performing sit-ups".

and facet joints of the spine. Analogy could be drawn to wearing out your tires by squealing them around sharp corners or bends in the road. Go for the highway mileage when it comes to exercising your spine. Rotating the trunk to perform a boxing punch is a partial and safe abbreviated motion.

Speaking of facet joints, more significance is now placed upon their contribution to low back pain. I have personally observed arthroscopic spine surgery which can cure certain types of low back pain by surgically desensitizing a single facet joint. (They are only about 1cm - 1½cm in diameter). With the patient fully awake and utilizing only xylocaine as anesthesia, the painful dime-sized facet joint was laser treated. Instantaneously, the grateful patient claimed complete relief while still lying on the operating table. This represents a miraculous scientific advancement, and clarification of the facet as a source of pain. As discs collapse the adjacent, micro-sized, facet joints are placed on a bind and certainly can become arthritic just like an injured hip or knee joint. Protect your back from crazy abnormal loading and twisting forces.

Chapter 14

Knee
(Figure 14-A)

Joe Namath, Danny Manning, Dick Butkus—knees, knees, knees. All too often this single joint is responsible for snuffing the illuminating career of the most promising and the most accomplished of athletes. A few years ago I attended a sports banquet featuring Dick Butkus as the after dinner speaker—arguably the toughest, meanest football player ever to lace up cleats. In order to continue smashing offensive linemen and attacking seemingly defenseless quarterbacks, his knees were multiply injected with cortisone on a weekly basis—for years. This regimen is now understood as an absolute taboo with our current knowledge of its devastating **long** term effects. Dick, quite honestly, confirmed that in his love for the sport, his trust in the team physician, and his team loyalty—he would have run through a brick wall if requested to do so. Not a person in the audience doubted his sincerity, iron-will, nor fearsome capability to accomplish such a request. Yet, this macho-man truly shed tears that night as he shared his feelings of betrayal at being "thrown away" by his team once his mighty knees fell apart. Despite his great loyalty to the team, he acknowledges that he was disallowed outside medical consultations and advice. He felt that his team doctor was transformed into an adversary working for "the company" rather than each athlete's health, performance, and longevity. Dick was asked to give his all, sacrifice his health each game, and donate his knees for life, with only unilateral loyalty. A sportsmedicine physician must never lose sight of an ultimate obligation toward each patient—not the team management. If an error is made, let it be

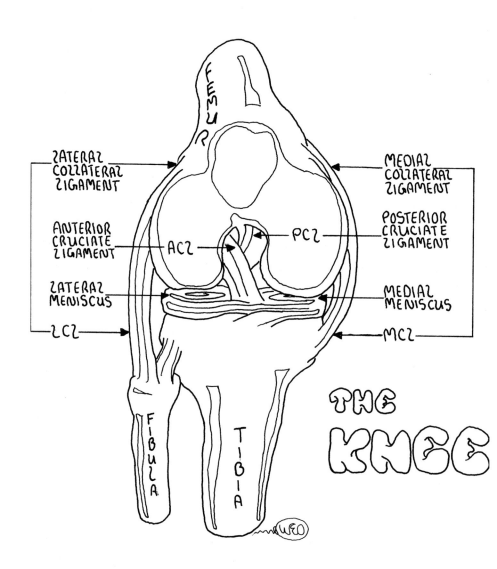

Figure 14-A: The knee

in fully advising each athlete of his options, and the short term/long term consequences. Then, let a properly informed athlete participate in decisions. Obviously, an overly competitive athlete must be restrained from participating if medical conditions warrant precautions and protection.

As a newly practicing sportsmedicine physician, I was long ago interviewed by a "gray hair" when being evaluated for orthopedic board certification. At that early stage of my career I was already employed as team physician for a professional soccer team. The examiner questioned me as to how I felt prepared to divulge critical decisions at such a larval stage of my career. I remain proud, satisfied, and committed with my then fortunate philosophy and answer, "I don't feel pressured to give edicts. My role is simply that of a teacher." I clearly, but thoroughly, informed my patient-athletes of their problems and choices and guided them in making any decisions. The heavy pressures, thus diffused, become shared in my kind of doctor-patient relationship. "I am not a dictator to be hated, debated, and overthrown, simply a teacher sharing my knowledge." I did get the green light on my boards and have tried to maintain that philosophy in all future relationships. Don't work for the team—work for each individual athlete! The doctor doesn't have to enforce decisions, the informed patient decides. After all, it is his body, not mine. Should strong advice be required, all that should suffice is, "If it was my knee …"

Dick Butkus routinely provided the first tackle and the last word. One classic encounter with an overmatched referee ended like this—after a heated on-field game dispute, the ref bit off more than he could chew as he carelessly told the meanest, toughest man in sport that a player shouldn't argue or this man in stripes would "bite his head off." Unfazed and unintimidated, Dick casually turned around as he walked to the sidelines and said, "If you do, you'll be the first human in history to have more brains in your gut than in your head."

Many "athletically-inclined" names have been created for this joint's many problems, i.e., runner's knee, jumper's knee, (Figure 14-B) and the devastating "terrible triad" designating a triple injury (two ligaments and a meniscus). The untreated anterior cruciate ligament injury has been significantly described as "the beginning of the end of the knee." I should know! Personally having experienced 3 surgeries on my left knee over a 22 year span and having operated on literally thousands of knee joints, I can claim familiarity to a fault. Living life as a "knee surgeon," I have counseled and treated many a devastated man or woman. But many were treated and feverishly adhered to a post injury or surgical program, rebounding to rejuvenated accomplishments. There is hope! But as grandmother said, "Prevention is the best cure." Runners, aerobic students, dancers, basketball players, each "pound the ground" in their search for fitness.

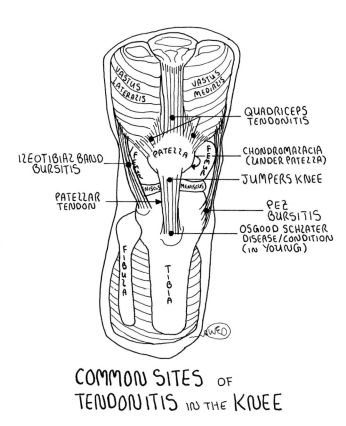

COMMON SITES OF TENDONITIS IN THE KNEE

Figure 14-B: Common sites of tendonitis about the knee

A scientifically designed "zone system" of aerobic boxing fitness allows "dealer's choice" in selecting the intensity placed on the lower extremity (legs), upper extremity (arms), and trunk. Optional boxing movements exercise the **lower extremities** in various maneuvers:

    1. Punching

    2. Bobbing and weaving

    3. Foot switching—a three minute Boxergenics™ drill

Why do I include **punching** when talking about leg exercising? The punching movement should not generate its power solely from the arms but quite significantly from the stored energy released by the torque and rotation of the trunk (i.e., abdominal muscles, low back muscles) and hips. The legs firmly anchor us to the ground allowing our properly positioned body to release its coiled springs (arms) which are poised to strike. Uncoordinated leg movements can stress the knee ligaments, meniscus, and joint surfaces.

Bobbing and weaving (partial squatting movements) tend to place more stress across the patella (kneecap) than other structures of the knee joint. These repetitive and classic "up and down" boxing motions can play havoc with a patella that already has seen its better days.

The **foot-switching** exercise is generally safe for most knee conditions unless your knee is "plain and simple" arthritic and worn out. This fitness exercise requires switching left foot forward position with a rapid right foot forward stance as your body remains stable, neither moving forward nor backward. This really drives up the training heart rate and warms up the body for more aggressive movements. Foot switching promotes rapid foot responses and body balance—agility. Don't bounce up and down during the foot-switching exercise. Your head and shoulders should stay level and at a constant height. These aren't jumping jacks. Work the foot pattern in a straight line if your knee is irritated. If you must compensate for underlying patella wear—don't bend your knees very much and don't piston up and down.

THE OFTEN INJURED MENISCUS

Patients over and over again express disbelief that signs of a torn meniscus arrive without a significant traumatic event. "I didn't do anything to tear it" they profess. "How can this happen? I was simply doing an exercise that I do every workout." "I don't remember hurting it." They forget all the soccer games, deep squats, basketball games, and long distance runs. My lecture always draws upon the example that—cars can be damaged either slowly (by gradual wear and tear forces) or suddenly in an accident—same with the knee joint. If one inappropriately bounces and twists many, many times over the years—the damaged and weakened tissues can finally tear through. One always questions—Why did my achy knee so suddenly get sore and lock up on me? The weak spot finally tore through! (Figure 14-C)

Maybe my FAN BELT theory may also help. How many travelers have been stopped in their car tracks as the engine overheats and a broken fan belt

PROGRESSION OF MENISCUS INJURY

NORMAL　　WEARING　　TORN

•FULL GO　　•ACHES　　•SWOLLEN
　　　　　　　　　　　•POPS
　　　　　　　　　　　•CATCHES
　　　　　　　　　　　•LOCKS UP

Figure 14-C: Progression of meniscus injury

becomes the culprit? We all understand that some inconspicuous fraying had to be present within an apparently functional fan belt before the tear occurred. It just happens. The disruption of functioning parts doesn't have to follow a major insult such as an auto accident or a 110°F summer drive. The meniscus can work reasonably well until an unnoticed twist or deep squat delivers the "coup-de-grace." We can't always peer back into our extensive, compulsive runner's log and pinpoint that one critical mistake. It may simply be related to many training miles, poor alignment, earlier injuries, or bad luck.

Study the four photographs that I obtained from various patients during surgery. The first indicates a normal smooth-edged meniscus. (Figure 14-D) Early "flap" tear in a professional basketball player is shown in the second photograph. (Figure 14-E) Photograph #3 displays a displaced, "balled-up," degenerated meniscus tear in a wrestler. (Figure 14-F) A displaced "bucket-handle" tear that is totally slid out-of-place and locking-up the knee in this martial artist is demonstrated in the fourth photo. (Figure 14-G)

The menisci can also acutely tear by sharp, sudden overloading forces impacted into a sharply flexed knee or rotational forces driven onto a weight-bearing knee. If one violently twists or rotates in an untimed movement, while throwing a punch or being dropped to the mat during a swift single-leg take down, a healthy part can tear. Keep your footwork and body movements coordinated, smooth, and adhering to the proper form. Ask your coach to critique.

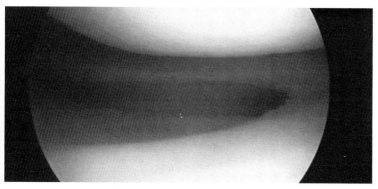

Figure 14-D:
Normal,
smooth-edged
meniscus

Figure 14-E:
Early flap tear

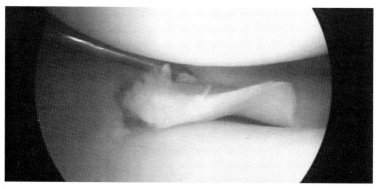

Figure 14-F:
Displaced,
"balled-up"
degenerated
meniscus tear

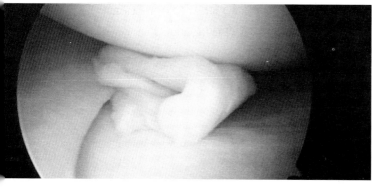

Figure 14-G:
Displaced
"bucket handle"
tear that has
totally slid out
of place and is
locking up the
knee

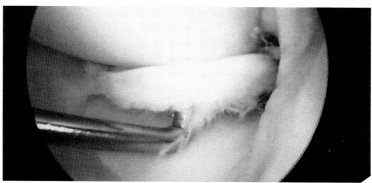

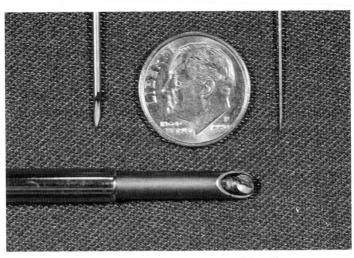

Figure 14-H: Arthroscope as compared to a dime

If you suddenly slip in class, on the soccer field, or on wet leaves in the parking lot, an acute tear may occur. Unfortunately even brand new cars can get in wrecks. It is not always possible to prevent accidents.

You can help yourself by recognizing common mechanical symptoms of a misshapen, torn meniscus. If your knee grinds, locks up, catches, pops, or swells, a torn meniscus is a distinct possibility. The meniscus is your shock absorber. A torn and displaced meniscus must be treated before that sliding tissue harms the other weight-bearing surfaces of your joint—actually creating permanent arthritis. Most will understand that grit must be removed from a bearing before it scratches the opposing bearing surfaces and "burns out" the bearing. Seek care if mechanical "happenings" alert you. Meniscus tears don't show up on plain x-rays so more sophisticated studies such as an MRI (Magnetic Resonance Imaging) must be performed to outline and confirm the tear. Dye studies are painful, invasive, old-fashioned, and no longer state-of-the-art. Eventually, arthroscopic surgery must be performed to remove or occasionally re-suture the mobile segment. See photograph of scope (at bottom of picture) comparing it to a dime. (Figure 14-H) The meniscus may be irreparably damaged or possess such a tenuous blood supply that the torn portion rarely heals—(Figure 14-I) thus it often requires removal (excision). You ask "Isn't it bad to remove an original part of the knee?" Yes, but I always explain it to my patients this way. "The best way to have your knee is the way God

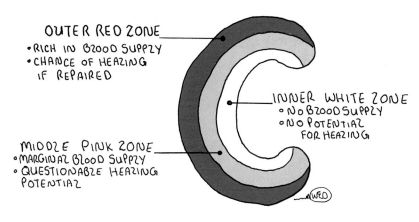

OUTER RED ZONE
•RICH IN BLOOD SUPPLY
•CHANCE OF HEALING
  IF REPAIRED

INNER WHITE ZONE
◦ NO BLOOD SUPPLY
◦ NO POTENTIAL
   FOR HEALING

MIDDLE PINK ZONE
◦MARGINAL BLOOD SUPPLY
◦ QUESTIONABLE HEALING
  POTENTIAL

(WED)

VASCULARITY of MENISCUS

Figure 14-I: Vascularity of meniscus

made it. The worst is to have a piece scratching the joint. The best compromise is to remove the damaged portion." Arthroscopic surgery is generally an out-patient procedure and only tape (steri-strips) or a single suture are utilized to close the 3 or 4 small incisions.

MENISCUS REPAIR

The best of all scenarios, when a meniscus does present as cleanly torn, is a repair. Repair opportunities remain limited for several reasons already mentioned. First, tenuous blood supply supports repair only if the tear occupies the more vascular outer rim. No blood, no healing! Secondly, the tear must be reasonably simple. A beat up, scraggly, chopped-up piece of tissue is best removed. Thirdly, the tear must lie in a position that is safely accessible to arthroscopic instrumentation. Certain tenuous locations endanger arteries and nerves living in the neighborhood whereas other accessible areas for repair are relatively easy targets. At this point in time, most doctors perform a rather low percentage of repairs compared to "trim-outs." We all hope that current and ongoing research in repair technique will simplify options. As it stands now, if your meniscus allows repair, a more prolonged time on crutches is recommended for protecting the healing tissue. Due to the fact that sutures are placed across repaired tissue, six weeks of limited activity is a must for your healing process to knit the torn ends together. The stitches don't heal the wound, you do! The sutures are only used to gather injured tissues closer together so that nature has a smaller gap to close. Sutures by themselves don't cause healing. You must allow injured tissues a fighting chance to proceed through their stages of repair. When a piece has been simply removed, the basic recovery only occupies several weeks for the knee to "quiet down" (both from the surgery and the pre-existing injury).

CHONDROMALACIA

If you hear or feel grinding noises as you:

1. Climb or descend stairs

2. Squat down

3. Straighten your knee while in a sitting position

they are probably symptomatic of a defective and injured articular cartilage layer under your patella. That diagnosis is "runner's knee" or chondromalacia, **chondro** means "cartilage" and **malacia** means "softening of"; thus— softening of the cartilaginous undersurface of your patella. This hyaline cartilage functions like a coating of formica on a wooden kitchen counter o enamel on a sink, creating a smooth, shiny, gliding surface. God gave us on ly one serving of this hyaline cartilage layer when we were born and we can' produce any more of it, even if it wears out. Sometimes arthroscopic surgery properly utilized, can shave down the irregular, frayed cartilage fragments See photo of chondromalacia and notice the frayed, irregular edges that ca

be smoothed and trimmed ("given a haircut") at surgery. (Figure 14-J) But remember, this surgery can allow great improvement, but it only removes damaged tissue. Science remains in its infancy in creating new tis-

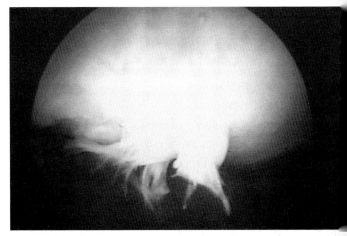

Figure 14-J: Chrondromalacia patella "Needing a haircut." Fraye irregular edges that can be smoothed and trimmed at surgery.

sue or synthesizing retreads. Currently, and under the proper surgical conditions, there exists the opportunity to surgically induce some lower quality (scar) fibrocartilage to plug these holes—similar to applying plastic wood compounds to fill defects versus the existence of real wood. New technology may allow the two-stage implantation of culture-grown hyaline cartilage cells into a properly prepared defect.

Great compressive forces travel across your patella during sports activities. For example, a compressive force 2 to 3 times one's body weight develops simply as we squat or travel down stair steps. Our patella works like a pulley system across the front of our knee. (Figure 14-K)

If you are harassed with symptoms of kneecap wear, your exercise future remains viable with certain modifications and compromises. Whereas classic aerobics, running, bicycling, and Stairmaster may be irritating; and soccer, basketball, hill running, and squatting may be harmful, creativity abounds for modified aerobic boxing workouts. This safer option applies because the exerciser refrains from bending his/her knees to any significant degree. Work harder to load up your arms and trunk. Minimize the depth of squatting as you bob and weave. Keeping knees relatively stiff limits exposure to excessive pressure. Do properly stretch the front of your thighs (quadriceps) during warm-up or cool-down to lessen the tension across the front of your knee.

PATELLA REHAB

A physical therapist can teach you exercises to restore the symmetric tone of the quadriceps muscle—a key in promoting and re-establishing the tracking of a patella. Kneecaps can "get out of alignment" and wear just like an improperly aligned or imbalanced tire tread on your car. Many mistakes are made when treating patellar injuries. Many a patient has sought my advice after inappropriate prior treatments. Their typical story is ... "My knee actually feels worse after I performed the exercises that were prescribed for me." The entire game plan should change once the patella is recognized as injured. Squats and full range of movement leg extensions (classic isotonic exercises) place too much pressure on the injured cells of a kneecap. Regular exercises only further beat up the knee. Essentially, only minimal movement or (isometric) limited arc routines are allowed.

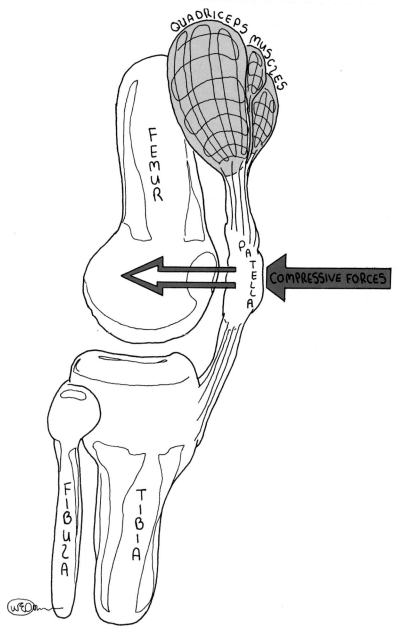

THE BODY PRODUCES COMPRESSIVE FORCES
2-3x BODY Wt. WHEN SQUATTING OR
CLIMBING STAIRS. THIS CAN BE MANY TIMES
GREATER WITH OTHER CHALLENGING SPORTS.

Figure 14-K: Compressive forces on patella

Matching areas of your kneecap and thigh articulate (rub) at varying angles of movement. The trick is to avoid loading the damaged tissue, yet exercising the quadriceps muscles so only the healthy surfaces of the patella make primary contact. (Figure 14-L, Figure 14-M, and Figure 14-N)

The fancy medical/rehabilitation term for these limited movements is isometric progressive resistance exercises (isometric p.r.e.'s).

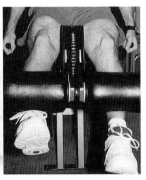 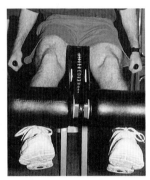 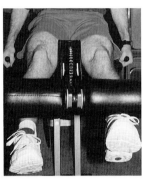

Figure 14-L: Isometric progressive resistance exercises recommended for patellar abnormalities

Figure 14-M: Isometric progressive resistance exercises recommended for patellar abnormalities

Figure 14-N: Isometric progressive resistance exercises recommended for patellar abnormalities

Jenny McConnell, a physical therapist from Australia, sophisticated a program that best isolates the muscle fibers responsible for the accurate tracking of the patella in its groove or notch. The application of these exercises and taping techniques necessitates a learning curve, so consult a sports therapist or physician for details. Initial therapy includes an early phase of biomechanically taping the knee. (Figure 14-O) This rehabilitation taping technique appears to be most effective and appropriate in assisting and supporting the early rehab efforts of knee exercises. The application of tape in a skillful manner is thought to unload sensitive contact areas of the articulations so that the introduction of rehab exercises accelerates recovery. Usually the need for taping decreases as symptomatic recovery progresses.

A good friend, expert martial arts instructor, sportsmedicine writer, and outstanding physician, Dr. Peter Lewis, resides in Melbourne, Australia. He personally suggests the application of these taping techniques to ease the occasional over-use injury. He relates that during an extensive, several day, long distance, group bicycle tour many discouraged, hurting participants requested his expertise one evening. That day's ride was rigorously demanding and took its toll. About to turn-in their helmets, gloves, and padded lycra shorts because of aching knees (patellar compression over-use), they asked their accompanying doc for help. Just the skilled application of

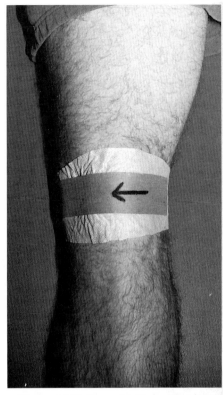

Figure 14-O: Jenny McConnell taping

McConnell taping transformed grimaces into smiles. The majority of those treated appreciatively confirmed the immediate effectiveness by painlessly peddling on the next day's ride. However, any long-term improvement requires a more comprehensive long-range plan.

Some braces can be useful in supporting the knee after injury. If your patella is poorly tracking, a brace with a circular cut-out hole and laterally located wedges may improve patella pressures.

ACL

In the early days of open reconstructive surgery (the 1950's and 1960's), the anterior cruciate ligament was not recognized as an important structure. When an injured knee was explored at surgery, some surgeons dismissed mentioning the ACL's state of health in their operative reports because it "served no major purpose." We now know better. The intricate activities of rapid starts and stops, quick cuts to the left or right, and jumping create tremendous torque

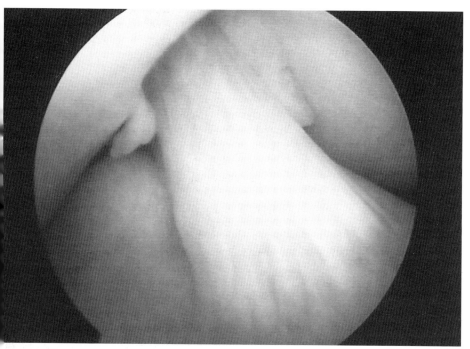

Figure 14-C: Normal, healthy ACL demonstrating normal fiber alignment

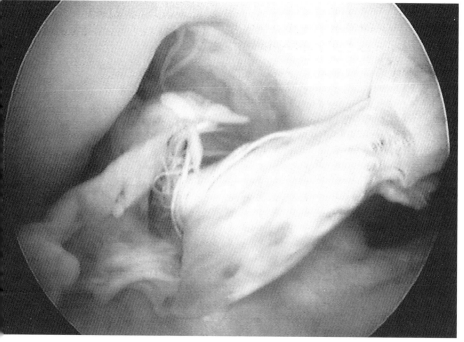

Figure 14-Q: Completely disrupted and displaced ACL tear

controlled by the ACL. This critical structure is considered the primary stabilizer for 3-dimensional movements of the knee. Our knee is accurately guided through a precisely smooth arc. See photo of normal, healthy ACL demonstrating normal fiber alignment. (Figure 14-P) A completely disrupted and displaced tear in a competitive martial artist is demonstrated in the second photo. (Figure 14-Q)

LACHMAN SIGN

Our understanding of these intricacies was catapulted into modern application, not within the hallowed halls of a major university but by a small town surgeon, Dr. Lachman. He treated many snow-skiers on winter pilgrimages to a small Western mountain resort. An intuitive, observant patient actually demonstrated to this doctor the giving away pattern that plagues the cruciate deficient athlete. Dr. Lachman was not only able to interpret the slipping and sliding symptoms but was then clever enough to design a physical exam test to reproduce these tell-tale shifts. (Figure 14-R, Figure 14-S Anterior drawer test, and Figure 14-T Lateral pivot shift test)

How do these "pivotal" injuries occur? Most commonly, you will have no one else to blame but yourself as non-contact injuries are responsible about 80% of the time. Snow skiing, itself, reportedly produces 100,000 new ACL tears per year in the United States. Soccer is not such a benign sport. While serving as team physician for a professional soccer team in the early eighties, I had occasion to reinspect our pre-season team photograph at season's end.

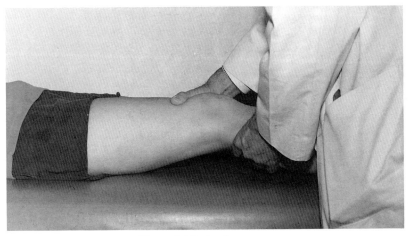

Figure 14-R: Lachman test

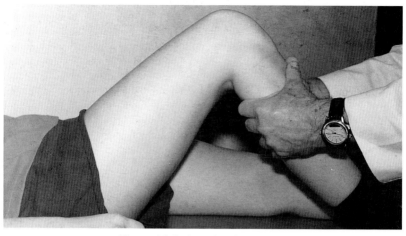

Figure 14-S: Anterior drawer test

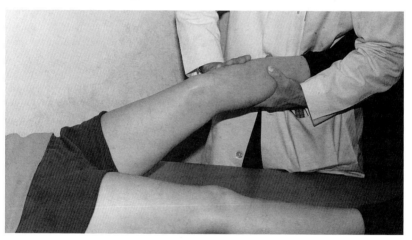

Figure 14-T: Lateral pivot shift test

By the last game, three of seventeen players had torn their ACL's. These 3 players were coincidentally standing next to each other during that photo. No, don't think that it's a virus! I was standing on the sidelines during a particular game and actually watching Miguel as he suddenly dropped to the ground. Alone, he was chasing the ball to the sidelines with the intention to turn it back onto the field of play before it went out of bounds. This sturdy, high intensity, seasoned veteran from South America had duplicated this move tens of thousands of times during his development. Somehow his timing was off and, without being touched by an opponent, over-rotated on his planted leg. The classic "pop" was felt and heard by this mid-fielder as he dropped like a stone.

He could not walk off the field and, of course, could not continue playing. Most individuals cannot "play on" with an ACL tear as compared to other more subtle injuries. We iced his knee but, despite this measure, he developed a large knee effusion (fluid in the joint) within several hours. Sometimes a knee will feel "locked" because strands of the ligament will flop into the joint blocking and binding up movement. My subsequent exams revealed a diagnostically excessive front-to-back laxity in his knee (Lachman's sign) and "jumping out of place" feeling when stressed movement was applied (lateral pivot shift). Miguel did agree to my recommendation for surgery which I performed several days later. He returned the next season as a starting mid-fielder. He phoned me 3 or 4 years later after his retirement. He was now in graduate school on the West Coast and had recently torn his **opposite** ACL during a recreational pick-up game.

Lynn, on the other hand, was a Karate instructor and high level National Team Tae Kwon Do competitor. She, likewise, had challenged her every arm and leg to the max during her fights. Having never been seriously injured, she was very tolerant of the bumps and bruises inherent in her sport. I remember her as a petite, red-headed, ball-of-fire whose intensity was not to be doubted. Her ACL was torn during the instruction of beginning level karate students. She simply jumped carelessly over one student who was lying on the mat, felt that "pop," and collapsed. The simplest of movements caught her knee in a twist for which she was not prepared. It is mind boggling to expect "a hop" to hobble an instructor who was so sophisticated in jumping, spinning, and flying kicks. I performed her reconstructive surgery and she returned to competition but withdrew after 1½ seasons to guard against re-injury to her re-built knee. Her outlet as an instructor, rather than as a competitor, was satisfying enough.

Clay was a 39 year old Aikido instructor. During a training session he was in the midst of lifting an opponent and starting to pivot for the throw. A practice-ending painful pop left him quite sure that something serious had occurred. As a seasoned competitor he was quite used to bumps, bruises, and pain, but knew that this injury required evaluation. He was examined in my office thirty-six hours later. Swelling of a moderately large amount ballooned his knee. The ability to squat was impossible due to the swelling and pain. The Lachman test, used to evaluate if the tibia (shin bone) will excessively move forward on the femur (thigh bone), was positive—showing laxity. He had torn his ACL. Fluid removal from his knee was not indicated as our exam was sufficient to confirm the problem.

One must understand that "fluid on the knee" (an effusion) is the **result** of a problem and not **the** problem. If you poke yourself in the eye, your eye will water. If you get grit in your eye, your eye will water. Simply wiping away the tears will not address the cause—grit in your eye. Likewise, simply drawing fluid off the knee will not treat the underlying condition. We must ultimately remove the grit, fix a torn meniscus or ligament, to provide a lasting cure. Occasionally we will withdraw fluid to temporarily relieve pressure, analyze for blood versus irritation fluid, or perform a laboratory search for signs of crystals (gout) or infection.

Clay did proceed to surgery for an arthroscopically assisted reconstruction of his ACL. (Figure 14-U) Some additional damage to the articular surfaces of his thigh bone had also occurred. The torque of his injury caused additional trauma as so frequently accompanies an ACL tear. Great effort was expend-

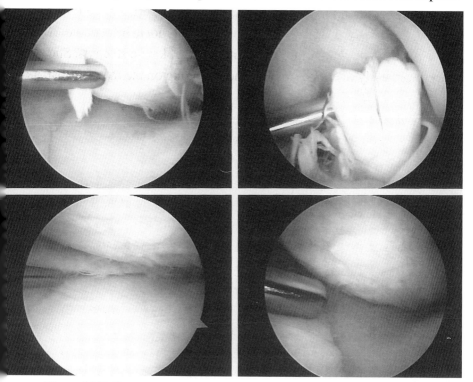

Figure 14-U: Post surgery arthroscopically assisted reconstruction of ACL

ed by him in his recovery and he is currently in a protected, limited activity, rehabilitation exercise mode.

Let's review the pattern—a sudden twist during acceleration or deceleration, followed by an audible or felt "pop." One's ability to walk is hindered, and fluid builds up within several hours. Locking of the knee may be present. A further exam would reveal blood in the knee rather than a more gradual build-up of clear joint fluid. Currently, we recommend that most young, active athletes undergo a reconstruction. I use the term reconstruction because we can't repair your original tissue with any confidence. Most torn cruciates are stretched-out and frayed beyond repair. Other ligaments or tendons around your knee can be safely removed and transferred into your knee as a substitute. Additionally, freeze dried or fresh frozen cadaver tendons are commonly acceptable sources of material. This surgery has progressed from open, multiple, long incisions to arthroscopically assisted procedures. I have "grown-up" as a knee surgeon while the parade of advances has marched forward. My initial and early patients had long incisions, drain tubes, days of hospitalization and long leg plaster casts worn for 6 weeks. Currently, incisions are minimal because of the arthroscope, and protected motion of the knee begins immediately or within a few days. Many times, walking is allowed as soon as muscle tone returns, pain is reasonable, motion is progressing, and swelling is subsiding. However, don't take this reconstructive procedure lightly. A major commitment of protection and physical therapy must parallel your surgeon's efforts. I like to advise my patients that the surgery is 50% of the job and their physical therapy efforts fully occupy the other one-half. This surgery will fail if the patient doesn't carry his share of the load. Although a rare athlete has played football six months after his ACL graft, 12 months is the safest time table to mentally program into your "hard drive." Why? Any tissue grafted into the center of your knee is initially void of circulation. It is in the grossest of terms—a piece of avascular, dead tissue. Over time, here comes that 12 months again, blood vessels grow into each end of the graft and carry with them new cells—"creeping substitution." Your body remakes the graft into its own new living ligament, slowly transforming itself by graduated stresses applied through physical therapy challenges. Consider the early graft as simply a trellis that roses will grow across or struts in a vineyard that are later entwined with grapes. Slowly controlled exercises strengthen the vine but be aware that quick, overpowering forces will tear apart the young green branches. Choose a great surgeon and latch onto a great physical therapist.

After all of that blood, sweat, tears, and effort, a specialized knee brace might be considered for high risk activities. Specialized braces for ligament tears are necessary. If an anterior cruciate ligament instability is your problem, only a $600.00+ brace is sophisticated enough to have a chance of stabilizing your knee. You are fooling yourself to buy inexpensive substitutes. Three dimensional forces are involved and only a hi-tech brace has a fighting chance to restrain your knee into its anatomic axis. Over-the-counter hinged braces are suitable for straight medial and lateral ligament sprains. Certainly consult a knee surgeon to sort out and identify which ligaments are responsible for your knee instability.

If you are (1) not engaged in sudden acceleration sports, (2) your knee does not pivot out of place, (3) you are older, and (4) no swelling occurs, then rehab and bracing only may suffice. Check in for exams every year or so. I have lost track of several patients who tore their ligaments, chose not to have surgery, and felt that they were doing o.k. One patient stated that he was regularly playing tennis so he reasoned that his knee had to be doing all right. He was wrong. Several years later he appeared for an office visit because his knee was clearly swollen (even to him). X-rays and exam revealed a very arthritic knee in a 27 year old businessman. We had lost touch and I had no chance to monitor his subtle symptoms. It is best to have a third party check you out once in a while. Nurturing parents don't recognize changes as they see their infant on an hourly and daily basis. It requires out-of-state grandparents and friends to occasionally appreciate the great changes in appearance. If you harbor a chronic injury, don't drift into nonchalance and procrastination. Seek medical guidance! As I mentioned earlier, a torn cruciate denies your knee a smooth, contoured arc of movement. In its absence the knee, either grossly or in thousands of mini-episodes (pivot shifts), jumps out of alignment and abrades other structures within the joint. If you live with an ACL-deficient-knee and also live an active life, one structure after another is sacrificed until you own a knee that is not worth fixing. Your old car is ready for the salvage dump rather than worthy of an alignment and tune-up. Don't treat yourself, you are not an unbiased judge.

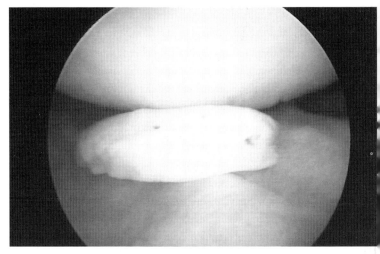

Figure 14-V-1: Loose body in the knee

LOOSE BODIES

Sometimes a piece of articular cartilage can break-off in the joint and
float freely. If the piece happens to
lodge in a weight-bearing area it can
also lock-up a joint. A small insignificant piece can actually continue to
grow as it floats around in joint fluid
which continues to nourish it. They are
easily removed at arthroscopy. (Figure
14-V-1 and Figure 14-V-2)

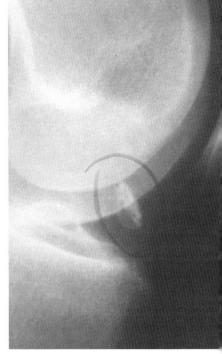

Figure 14-V-2: Loose body in the knee

ARTHRITIS

If your doctor finds arthritis (a loss of the articular hyaline cartilage or "formica" that coats your joints) he/she may perform surgical techniques that promote the ingrowth of "scar" cartilage. This replacing **fibrocartilage** is a substitute material that can improve our function but lacks the durability of the original product **hyaline cartilage.** Think of fibrocartilage as a substitute—a filler that can "patch-over" defects. Six weeks of partial weight-bearing—after appropriate surgical procedures—and careful protection give you the best odds for its fullest formation. Some patients are good at making scar cartilage and others never fill-in the gaps. Fibrocartilage best plugs small isolated defects but can't adhere to and re-surface an extensively burnt-out knee. Even greater hope for restoration of isolated defects on joint surfaces appears on the horizon. I am one of a restricted group of doctors trained to perform an innovative procedure whereby an individual patient's cultured cartilage cells are reimplanted, as a paste, onto a properly prepared joint defect. Researchers in Sweden initiated research supporting the concept that cartilage cells can be grown in a lab in quantities sufficient enough to re-coat isolated defects in injured joints. This method spearheads a "new wave" direction in reparative procedures. Total knee replacement with plastic and metal components remains a God-send to end-stage patients but is **not** compatible with sports activities.

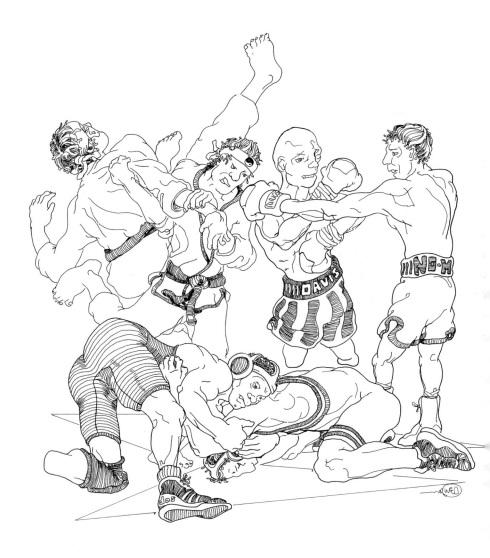

Chapter 15

Leg

STRESS FRACTURES

Is there any He-man or Wonder Woman among you that can tear a wire clothes hanger in-half with a brutal outburst of raw power and energy? I doubt not. I do guarantee, however, that I could accomplish this monumental task by prompting any youthful volunteer to bend that same wire back and forth 60 times preceding that now wimpy feat. I have just described the basis of a stress fracture. Repeated and multiple minute traumas to an over-stressed bone can overpower our living tissues ability to keep up with the minute-to-minute constant repair process that our body monitors. Bone is truly a living tissue and not an amorphous hunk of concrete-like calcium. The leg bone that you are standing on at this instant is not the leg bone that you jogged upon or bicycled with one year ago—nearly every cell has been updated and replaced. If you overpower this process with "too much—too soon" the break-down in stress points will out-strip the remarkable repair and reinforcement process. Runners get stress fractures because their foot, ankle, leg (tibia and fibula), thigh, hip, or pelvis was never given the R & R—rest and recuperation (**relative rest**) needed. Generally, running in excess of 20 miles per week makes you an at-risk statistic. Boxergenics™, by creating a zone system of shared exercise responsibility, can creatively dissipate the forces by ⅓ challenges to each functioning body unit—upper extremities, trunk, and lower extremities.

X-rays will often fail to identify an early stress fracture. The insult is delivered on such a microscopic level that the weakened bone often fails to appear

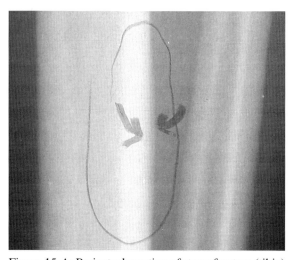

Figure 15-A: Periosteal reaction of stress fracture (tibia)

as a visible crack on early x-ray. The bone cells may not have had time to mount a visible healing response. Go back to our hanger example. At the 35th bend the paint on the hanger remains intact and only a microscopic exam would reveal disruption of the internal metal bonds. Visual inspection might show no gross defects. In living tissue after 3 to 6 weeks, a doctor might begin to spot subtle healing responses in the area of the injury. Often we never see the actual crack, only the callous (glue, solder, or weld) of new bone. (Figures 15-A and 15-B) A bone scan is the most accurate, cost-effective, (approximately $750.00) early test if confirmatory evidence is required and necessary. But don't tempt fate. Pushed too far—you'll get the opportunity to hear the crack, see your deformity, and experience the damp, moldy, smelly confinement of a cast. I have actually witnessed the progression of an easy-to-manage tibia stress injury into a full blown broken-in-half fracture. A young lady, a junior in high school, was preparing for the spring track season as the late winter winds whistled and snow still fell. The enthusiastic shut-in ran on the unyielding concrete hallways of her school and the tight

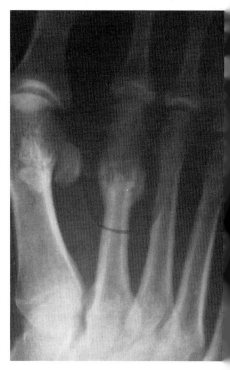

Figure 15-B: Metatarsal callous as shown on x-ray of a healing stress fracture

small-circle course of the gymnasium. Overuse was predictable. An accidental slip down the school steps created an angulated, full-blown, set-that-fracture, long-leg-cast-for-three-months type of situation. The break occurred exactly through the previously diagnosed, minimally positive x-ray, stress area. Something easy was made difficult! If caught early, just a slow down in activity or switch to ALTERNATIVE activity would have done the job. Why not be smart and use the ALTERNATIVES inherent in cross-training from the get-go? Spread out the stress, share the load!

Should stress injury develop, don't fight it. Realize it and admit a temporary surrender and truce. **A stress fracture will always, always win.** Your body will shut down that injured part by pain and disuse until it is satisfied that the healing has advanced to a tolerable level.

Many times the problem is obvious and classic enough to simply incorporate the history and exam together for a clinical diagnosis. Let your doctor's experience dictate the need for additional studies and the need to cut down on activity. Remember, I said **cut down.** Rarely is absolute rest or a cast necessary. The severity of treatment depends upon how soon the problem is identified and respected. Without a doubt a stitch in time saves—well—time.

MEDIAL TIBIAL STRESS SYNDROME (SHIN SPLINTS)

Repeated pounding may injure a bone causing a **stress fracture** but micro-trauma can also tear away at the attachment of muscles onto bone causing **medial tibial stress syndrome.** The backside of the tibia (shin, leg) bone is flat and an attachment site for calf and leg muscle. Micro-tearing of these hook-ups can translate into the ache and leg sensitivity that hampers or halts the training of a dancer, aerobics instructor, soccer player, or runner. Many principles of the stress fracture example might also apply so that the two diagnoses may appear as twins, one concentrated to bone (stress fracture) and the other related to muscle/tendon (shin splints). The bone injury tends to be isolated to a pinpoint area, whereas the medial tibial stress syndrome will be spread out over several inches. With medial tibial stress syndrome x-rays remain negative while a bone scan shows uptake over a large but mildly intense area. The cure for both is essentially the same. **RELATIVE REST.** Besides over-training, other causes can be leg length inequality (one leg longer than the other so that we are rocking the boat), excessive pronation (poor foot posture where the foot rolls inward and unsupported), tight calf muscles, improper shoes (worn out and in need of being dumped in the garbage can), poor alignment of the legs (such as bow-legged or knock-kneed), and poor exercise technique. See a podiatrist or sportsmedicine trained doctor for a "whole body" evaluation. One can't just look at the sore spot and draw accurate conclusions. Don't forget to analyze the "big picture" when worried about details ... as many compulsive exercisers tend to do. The doctor has to stay cool, circumspect and analyze all factors, not just focus on the date of the upcoming marathon that you **must** run!

TREATMENT

If an imbalance of the leg muscle strength occurs, posterior tibial stress syndrome may result. Usually the front or anterior muscles in the shin are weak. A simple and practical exercise is called "heel walking." With a pair of shoes on to pad your feet, start walking around the room **on** your heels with toes pointing up. Walk for about 2 or 3 minutes. You will feel the "burn" in the exercised muscles. This emphasis will balance the dorsiflexors (frontal muscles) with respect to the more usually exercised plantar flexors (calf muscles). It goes without saying that other mechanical or training errors must be simultaneously corrected.

COMPARTMENT SYNDROME

Have you ever been imprisoned within a pair of new shoes that were so tight that:

(1) Every step felt like your tender little toe was destined to become a raw bleeding stump?

(2) Each successive beat of your heart was cascading downward as rapids into your feet?

(3) You couldn't wait to kick off your shoes and go barefoot however inappropriate or unmannerly?

This brief short story provides some insight into the pressure characteristics of a tight tissue compartment within the leg.

First, a brief anatomy lesson. The leg or calf area is composed of 4 separate muscle groups—each wrapped in a firm, taut, unyielding covering called fascia. A great example is that of a hot dog or Polish sausage — contents circumferentially packed and stuffed within a membranous wrap. (Figure 15-C) Each compartment is a little community all unto its own with tendons, muscles, nerves, arteries (high pressure vessels) and veins (low pressure vessels). Certain individuals, either by inheritance (luck of the draw) or injury (just plain bad luck),

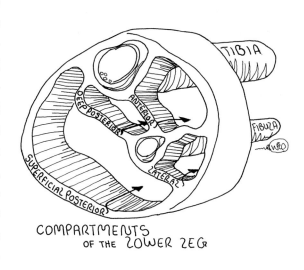

COMPARTMENTS OF THE LOWER LEG

Figure 15-C: Compartments of the leg

possess potentially tight compartments. Too much sausage meat has been stuffed into their wrapper.

As we all know, exercise dramatically increases the blood flow to our muscles. Body builders fully take advantage of this physiologic response by intensely exercising just before their posing competitions to "pump up" their physique. As arterial blood is pumped into a compartment, muscle engorgement occurs and the pressure of the compartment increases. A critical state is pathologically reached if there is too much engorged muscle stuffed into too tight a sheath. An excessively elevated pressure blocks the outflow of the low pressure venous drainage, i.e., more people are getting stuffed into a crowded room with no chance to maneuver and leave by the exit doors. As panic sets in, the condition rapidly deteriorates. Muscles and nerves, which are very sensitive to pressure, become choked and die if enveloped into the extreme situation. I have treated a soccer player who was kicked in the leg, and many auto accident victims with broken legs, who required emergency surgery to split open their fascia compartments thus allowing the tissues to breathe … surgery necessary to abruptly halt the vicious injury-precipitated cycle of POINT A injury and bleeding causing POINT B swelling. If continued, the events lead to more pressure, more swelling, more pressure, and finally tissue death. (Figure 15-D)

Aerobic exercisers or runners don't enter the syndrome because of injury but subtly and chronically enter the syndrome at Point B. They can escape the vicious cycle by stopping their activity, resting for 2 - 10 minutes, and allowing the swollen pumped-up muscles to drain.

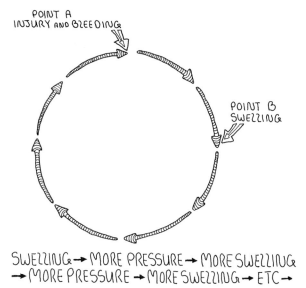

Figure 15-D: Vicious cycle of compartment syndrome

Kevin was a classic example. Although he had played soccer in the Select category for many years, it was not until his junior year in high school that his "leg endurance" became a problem. He could run and compete vigorously at "full-go" for only 12 - 15 minutes. As playing time and effort increased—a dull ache was more apparent in his leg—a tingling or numbness traveled into his foot. His muscles soon throbbed with the build up of lactic acid and other waste products. Earlier in the season a short rest would suffice to restore his speed and endurance. This defenseman sought my medical advice when it became clear that he spent more time on the bench protecting his leg than on the field defending his goal. Pressure studies by needle exam confirmed readings above 30mm Hg at rest and more dangerously elevated readings after a trial run. Surgery was performed as an out-patient, and he resumed full leadership as captain his senior year.

There are very few exercise options available to prevent and cure the symptoms. No particular stretch can physically expand the tough, thick fascia which envelops the compartments.

Chapter 16

Foot

ACHILLES TENDON TEARS

Although not often occurring in young, active, competitive athletes, athletic catastrophe becomes the best description when an Achilles tendon does tear. The most likely candidate suits a man in his 40's or 50's involved in a vigorous stop-start, jumping sport. Karate participants who spar are candidates. Routine class participation is not a high risk activity.

37 year old Aikido instructor, Aaron, was directing a 3-on-1 drill during a training class Thursday evening. This exercise teaches one to direct then re-direct his skill and energies against multiple attacking opponents. As he was accelerating in his spinning movement from aggressor #2 toward #3, his momentum was suddenly halted as #3 stepped onto his heel. The combination of suddenly halted acceleration and push-off caused his Achilles tendon to suddenly and thoroughly tear. A noticeable "pop" and immediate loss of function allowed no room for doubt or "let me shake it off a minute" thinking. Aaron knew that he was down for the count. His accumulated experience in motorcycle racing, martial arts, and rock climbing established a firm baseline from which to "know" his body. He recognized the seriousness and immediacy of his injury and traveled with his entourage to the emergency room where I met him. The reality is that the injured athlete generated the actual damaging forces internally and by his own doing. It was only the flow of events provided by opponents that negatively changed the timing for the contracting calf muscle.

Many other patients fail to immediately recognize the implications of this injury. It actually hurts less than one would expect. Many extensive ankle sprains will cause more pain and reaction than the sometimes reasonably isolated swelling of this major tendon rupture. In my experience, many patients have hobbled into the office one or two days later under the impression that they "sprained their ankle," "pulled my calf muscle," or "my foot doesn't work." They imagined some sort of ankle sprain. If you hear or feel a pop in your lower calf and cannot perform a toe raise, seek a sports physician. Early Greek mythology immortalized this major link between the calf muscle and the foot. The great warrior Achilles was rendered totally harmless when this structure was severed by his enemy's sword.

The Achilles tendon is the largest single tendon in the body with a rope-like density. Massive forces are generated during the acts of sprinting and jumping. Because it is so thick, the inner strands of tissue remain somewhat remote from an adequately penetrating blood supply and are disadvantaged for healing an injury. That's why Achilles tendonitis and tears heal so stubbornly. The body can't fully supply nutritional factors to the injured cells.

Aaron's story does typify many facets of this injury. Most of my patients were involved in tennis or basketball at their time of injury. Usually the patients have noticed very few warning signs or signals. Most are completely surprised, or should I say shocked, at the sudden, unexpected casualty. Some classic descriptions have been shared by patients.

One tennis player swore that some secretive sniper shot him in the calf as he lunged for an unreachable return. He heard the pop. A second later this patient nearly attacked his doubles partner accused of whacking him in the heel with a tennis racquet out of revenge for a missed shot. I'm happy to report that he was incapable of catching his innocent partner. An attorney friend tore his during a rugby match. One of my good friends from medical school tore both of his tendons over a 3 year span before his wife issued a forced retirement from his church basketball career.

Most tears occur within the tendon itself and not where the tendon attaches into the muscular portion of the calf (this area has a much better blood supply). At surgery the tears always appear irregular and mop-ended. When this "rope" finally frays through, the strands tear very irregularly as compared to a rope that is decisively sliced by a knife.

Two options for recovery exist—non-surgical and surgical. Don't confusingly relate these terms to conservative and non-conservative choices of treatment. Just because one option entails an incision, don't assume that your other choices are categorized into the conservative, easy, assured, painless pathway. I suggest that in this set of circumstances a surgical approach **may** actually prove to be your conservative alternative. When a complete, haphazard tear of the Achilles tendon occurs, (and most are complete) simply casting the leg doesn't in any way guarantee that the torn ends make contact with each other. With casting treatment, one can only hope that scar will fill-in the gaps. Additionally, the healed area doesn't assume the same mechanical tension as original anatomy planned. Many studies have confirmed that after treatment by casting, your ability to jump and regain power, is forever diminished. Only through open surgical placement of the tendon's "mop ends" will one arrive at a condition closer to the way God originally designed things. We surgeons simply attempt to restore the anatomy. Some controversy may exist with regard to proper treatment options. I strongly favor a surgical approach for 3 reasons:

1. I personally know 2 doctors who chose to have their injury treated in a cast for months rather than submit to the knife. One individual was chairman of the Department of Orthopaedic Surgery at a very prestigious hospital and training program. Another was chairman of the Pathology Department at a major referral hospital. Each limped about in a cast and on crutches for months before expected recovery. Each suffered a re-tear and subsequent surgery. They wasted tremendous effort and time.

2. At each of my surgical repairs, I am impressed, without exception, at the distance

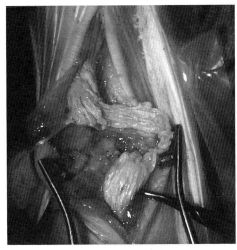

Figure 16-A: Torn achilles tendon at surgery

between the two torn ends. The gap usually measures one or two inches. The calf muscle is a powerful muscle which, when untethered, contracts with the spring of a window shade briskly snapped. There is no way that competent scar can fill the gap. One must also realize that such an injury is not a clean tear but appears more as the ends of 2 mops. (Figure 16-A and Figure 16-B) Only deliberate and purposeful surgical reattachment will assure some semblance of restored order.

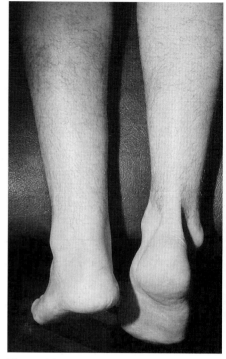

Figure 16-B: Patient with torn achilles tendon

3. Two groups of patients, surgical and casted, have been tested. The standing broad jump was utilized as a measure of regained strength and function. The surgically repaired patients dominated in this comparison of recovery.

After surgery, you will need cast protection for about eight (8) weeks, but during that eight weeks a series of casts may progress you towards an improved foot and ankle position within each cast. Some type of heel lift is recommended for several weeks after casting to keep pressure off the repair. During rehab, work for range of motion first and then concentrate on calf strength. If you rely upon a good physical therapist for this guidance, your chance of re-tear will be rather small. Complete recovery with full confidence takes eight or twelve months. If you choose the non-surgical casting route, your "down time" in casts must be a bit longer and more conservative. Your chance of re-rupture is greater. Therefore recognize the injury, seek an experienced physician, and realize that recovery will demand nearly one year for a confident return to athletics.

Even with a surgical cast still present on his leg, Aaron was able to partic-ipate in certain martial arts drills and classes as early as four weeks post surgery. He rode an exercise bicycle at four weeks using his good foot to main-tain some cardiovascular fitness and "keep his head clear." An upper body, trunk, and good leg weight training program were instituted at about three weeks post-op.

* **IMPORTANT NOTE:** Isolated but painful partial tears of the actual calf muscle do occur frequently in athletes. A similar mechanism—poorly timed lengthening of a poorly coordinated muscle contraction—can cause a small portion of the medial (inside) head of the gastrocnemius (calf muscle) to pop and tear. This hurts severely, cramps, swells, and bruises the leg. Crutches, elevation, ice, and anti-inflammatories are needed for significant symptoms. If reactive edema occurs in that foot, Jobst compressive machines used by physical therapists and prescribed supportive stockings can prevent the com-plication of phlebitis. If swelling and immobility are great, I recommend one or two aspirin tablets per day to lessen the chance of blood clots. Let your sports physician be your guide. The good news is—only a minor portion of the calf muscle usually tears. Once you are over the insult in one to three weeks, full function can be restored. Remember, the only way we heal back together again is by SCAR. Always participate in a properly supervised and executed stretching and warm-up program to promote proper alignment and length of that newly deposited healing scar. Don't set yourself up for repeat injuries by mistake after mistake or insult upon insult.

ACHILLES TENDONITIS

Achilles tendonitis is an inflammation and break-down of the very sub-stantial Achilles tendon as it attaches into our heel bone (calcaneus). The calf muscles provide push-off power to the foot, allowing us to rise up onto our toes in sprinting and jumping. If not hooked-up properly, a slap-stick Vaudeville-type gait results. The Achilles tendon (Figure 16-C) is the primary link between the calf muscles and the ability to point the foot downward.

Over-use of this tendon either by running, repeated jumping, or repeti-tive motions such as step aerobics or NordicTrack, can fatigue and fray the tendon fibers. I recently treated a 47 year old avid step aerobics participant

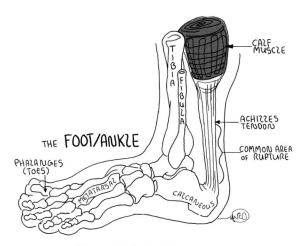

Figure 16-C: Achilles tendon

who noticed increasing "stiffness" and aching in his calf and ankle. After several months—a definite bulge was visible in his Achilles tendon. The conservative, non-surgical approach is producing some progress, but he can no longer attend lower body aerobic classes and may ultimately not escape the knife. I have operated on these chronic injuries and witnessed the change in appearance and texture of the central core of tissue within the tendon. Being such a massive and thick tendon limits the ability of blood to penetrate the central strands of this thick rope. (Figure 16-D) Injury degenerates the central segments and the resulting scarring thickens the tissue into a visible bulge. Symptoms include pain-after-activity, increasing local tenderness, and visible bulging. Treatment must include the self-discipline to cease the offending movements and to emphasize alternative exercise—a plan perfectly suited to aerobic boxing.

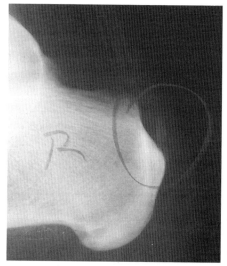

Figure 16-D: X-ray of achilles tendon calcification

- Use the trunks, arms, and hands more.

- Stretch the calf muscle more thoroughly and frequently throughout the day.

- Place a small heel lift into both shoes to remove constant tension on the injured area.

- Ice frequently.

- Ultrasound treatments by a physical therapist can help.

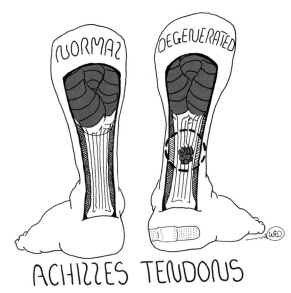

ACHILLES TENDONS

Figure 16-E: Achilles tendon degeneration

- Do not allow cortisone to be injected into this area. It can hasten rupture!

- Anti-inflammatory medicines may partially help, but because we are dealing with a mechanical problem, we more readily respond to mechanical cures than chemical cures.

- These areas of wear can abruptly tear apart requiring the need for urgent surgical repair. (Figure 16-E)

- Persistent cases require a surgeon to open the tendon and surgically remove the avascular, dead, necrotic center and then mend the outer fibers.

FOOT

The relative importance of feet was explicitly expressed on two signs clearly prominent during a visit to my friendly podiatrist's office:

1. "WHEN YOU HAVE A HEADACHE—YOUR HEAD HURTS. WHEN YOUR FEET HURT—YOU HURT ALL OVER." And

2. "THE AGONY OF DA FEET."

There is no pussy-footing around the fact that the combat arts require us to locate and position the body where the arms can be effective. Our feet propel us there. Aerobic boxing provides the distinct advantage that, should our legs falter, our arms can pick-up the exercise slack.

HEEL SPURS

Each and every time we take a step, our arch ligament tightens like a taut steel band. Examine your own foot. Keep weight off your foot as you sit and cross your leg. In this position you can not readily palpate much of an arch ligament. Put weight on your foot and a probing finger can now feel the taut band forming in the arch. The arch ligaments and muscle attachments form a sling across the bottom of our foot. If one bounces up and down with high impact aerobic movements upon an unyielding surface, our "foot 'spring' gets sprung." Small microscopic tears occur, just as Achilles tendonitis or tennis elbow. If your foot rolls in (pronates) excessively, microscopic tearing can also result. Many athletes label this heel soreness as a "stone bruise" or "heel spur" because it is so localized. "Heel spur" is a misnomer as there may be no relationship to any x-ray findings of our bone structures.

Yes, bone outgrowths called spurs may form in response to these injurious forces. But the basic pathology resides in the ligament damage. The bone spur forms in response to the stimulus of damaging forces as our body attempts to compensate in some manner. (Figure 16-F) In the old days of surgical management, the recommended treatment was to go in and resect (cut out) the bone spur. OK, it worked. But in cutting out the spur, the surgeon was also simultaneously releasing the offending tendon (which was really the true bad guy). The surgery performed on the neighboring structure actually vanquished the true villain with the same bang of the chisel. I usually remove the spur while I am performing the associated corrective surgery.

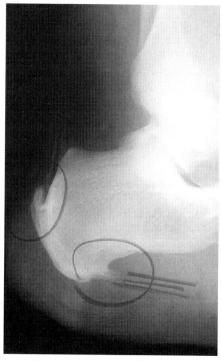

Figure 16-F: X-ray of heel spur

Many people whose feet are x-rayed for some unrelated purpose, i.e., ankle sprain, may show big old heel spurs and the patient may never have sensed any heel pain in their life. Other patients with serious pain and many months of failed treatment attempts may not demonstrate even the earliest hint of a baby spur. We recognize this problem as "soft tissue" in origin. Who can get it? Generally symptoms strike an individual with either a high arched foot or the other extreme—a flat foot. Quite often this athlete may excessively pronate (roll inward) on his/her foot.

Treatment plans should include the following:

• Avoid repetitive weight-bearing over-use movements. Are you getting the point by now? The treatment of **OVER-USE** injury must include some **UNDER-USE.**

• See a physical therapist, podiatrist, or athletic trainer for advice on foot exercises (yes, there are such exercises) and calf stretching.

• Anti-inflammatories can help a little (only a little).

• Physical therapy modalities, i.e., ultrasound or iontophoresis.

• Injections of cortisone by a sportsmedicine specialist. NOTE: Cortisone can be safely given in this area. Even if the cortisone caused the tissues to tear, the result is no different than our goal at surgery of releasing the tight tissues.

• Heel pads come in many sizes and configurations. The most effective style includes a soft spot of very forgiving silicone material positioned in the center of the heel region. (Figure 16-G)

• The ultimate biomechanical cure is an ORTHOTIC. An orthotic is not

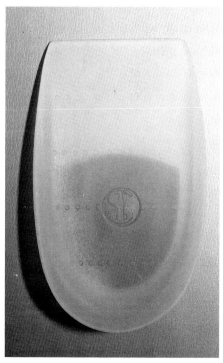

Figure 16-G: Silastic heel pad for heel spur (soft spot)

just a fancy, expensive, hand-made arch support. Correctly designed, an orthotic is a cast of the sole of the foot created WHILE THE FOOT IS POSITIONED BY THE DOCTOR IN ITS ANATOMICALLY NEUTRAL POSITION. Don't be fooled by pseudo-experts who ask you to stand fully weight-bearing on a measuring device. You are simply then paying big money for an "arch support." Arch supports simply fit the arch. A true orthotic demands that the bones of the foot are maneuvered into the anatomically preferred neutral stance rather than the collapsed shape of a foot in trouble. Once the proper cast is made, wedges (posts) are incorporated to prevent the foot from rolling in and out with every step. Without the troublesome rock and roll motion, your arch ligaments gain a fighting chance to heal.

• Occasionally surgery is performed to partially cut and release the arch ligament allowing it to retract, scar-in, and assume a more relaxed position. Although not a perfect procedure it is reasonably effective and most patients are happy with the results when more conservative techniques have failed.

Cortisone injections should be administered only occasionally. My applied advice is "3 strikes and you're out." If 3 injections spread out over 5 or 6 months (and no sooner than 4-6 weeks apart) don't work then 8 or 10 shots won't work either. The needle should preferably enter from the medial or inside area of your heel. (Figure 16-H) There is no reason to penetrate through the tough and important weight-bearing surface of your heel. The shot is much more painful if aimed through the bottom surface of the

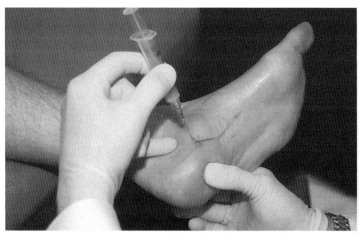

Figure 16-H: Heel injection entering inside area of heel

heel. Always demand a thorough and sterile cleansing of the injection site. An infection is a disaster.

A sad experience I shall not forget was the case of a hard working, self supporting, middle-aged waitress. She had been injected in the heel by another doctor 3 or 4 weeks prior to her consultation with me. The doctor didn't thoroughly cleanse the heel except with a casual alcohol wipe and her unrelenting pain and inability to walk signaled infection. Her visits with me soon confirmed an established heel bone infection. I recommended surgery and begrudgingly opened her heel widely with a 2 inch incision. Pus came rolling out as I scooped out a large portion of soft, dead heel bone. She eventually healed after several operations, I.V. antibiotics, and nearly 1 year of lost employment. Infections are very rare but a true disaster. Shots are 99.5% safe but must always be respected for their occasional side effects and risks. Consider every injection you receive, a "mini-operation."

FRACTURES OF THE ANKLE

Max Coats, a specialist in Shoot Fighting and Muay Tai, sponsored Bart Vale, then reigning world champion, as the guest instructor for a large seminar. Max, a highly skilled practitioner, was caught off guard when Bart performed a foot-sweep take-down as part of the demonstration. Full power was not critical to a teaching experience, especially since Max was sponsoring and funding his guest, Bart.

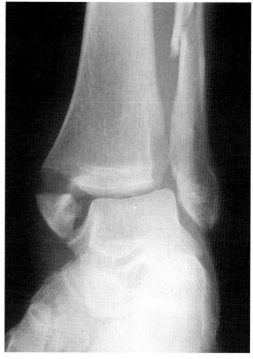

Max's foot stuck to the mat as Bart's 260-pound frame continued forward. The obvious pain and deformity delivered Max and his entourage to the emergency room where this x-ray of a broken, displaced ankle was

Figure 16-I: X-ray of broken, displaced ankle

obtained. (Figure 16-I) I took Max to surgery where the x-ray demonstrating the necessary plates and screws was obtained. (Figure 16-J) Max was extremely dedicated to his post-injury rehabilitation and continues to teach, fully active and competitive, having been granted an exclusively endorsed Gracie Jiu-Jitsu School.

ANKLE SPRAIN

First of all, get one concept straight. A sprain, any type of sprain, is a tear (maybe microscopic, but a tear just the same). Sprains (ligament tears) are graded or classified as I (mild), II (moderate), and III (severe).

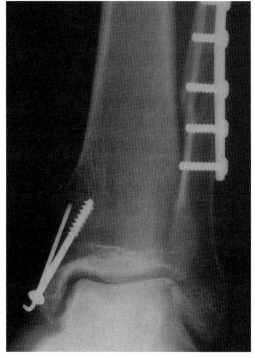

Figure 16-J: X-ray showing necessary plates and screws implanted during surgery

The problem is all the same, only varying by degree. (Figure 16-K) When one "turns-over" the ankle and hears or feels a "pop"—that "pop" represents fibers of your ligament tearing. Ligaments are living tissues and need a blood supply to exist. Bleeding into the surrounding tissues is natural as the torn ends of the ligament leak.

SWELLING

Nature designed our blood vessels (veins, arteries, capillaries, etc.) to bathe our miraculous complexity of cells with the fluids and nutrients that the ocean environment provided when early "mankind" was but a 2 or 3 cell blob floating in an ocean. As we became more and more complex creatures of God, a circulatory system developed to penetrate and nourish each expanding layer and organ. Our "ocean environment" blood has a high salt content that was meant to remain within its highways and byways. If blood escapes into surrounding tissues, a state of inflammation ensues and we recognize that as "swelling" and "pain." So, several hours after a sprained ankle, we notice the ankle puffing up and getting stiff. The rapid application of ice (for HEAVEN'S SAKE NOT HEAT) will limit the amount of bleeding and subsequent inflammatory response. Many times in my sportsmedicine practice I have recognized serious sprains with less swelling than I expected for the amount of tissue injury. A knowledgeable jock knew to apply ice. On the other hand, a fairly minor degree of tearing has presented itself as

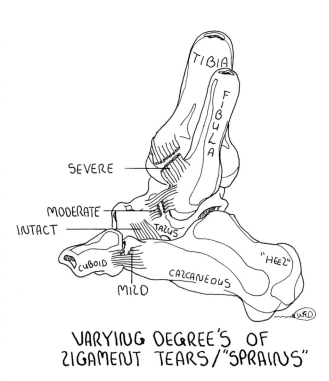

VARYING DEGREE'S OF ZIGAMENT TEARS / "SPRAINS"

Figure 16-K: Ligament tears — "sprains"

an ankle big and round as a stuffed sausage. You got it! Grandmother told him to go soak in hot water and epsom salts. What a setback! Misinformed coaches might pretend to be modern and prematurely misuse that expensive whirlpool sitting in the corner of the training room. The thinking is, "We may as well use it—it's paid for!" Not only is the heat a killer, but hanging the foot downward too soon after trauma only adds insult to injury.

Retreat to the knowledgeable trainer's recipe. R-I-C-E. Rest, ice, compression, elevation. Heat is useful only after the angriness resolves and stiffness primarily remains. In most athletic situations it may be 5 to 10 days before heat will not be a disadvantage. If one's reasoning for the use of heat includes the bringing of healing blood to the area, I'll give two thoughts. First of all, because of the tearing of tissues, too much blood floods the area initially. Secondly, ice does accomplish increased circulation to the wound, as a secondary effect. Think back. Once you remove an ice pack from your skin, don't you observe a pinkish flush to the skin? So, stick with ice until all initial warmth and irritation of the injury have been reduced, leaving only a stiffness that must be resolved. Ice also relieves the pain of an injury. If the local area is numbed by the coldness, you hurt less and less muscle spasm is created. I prefer plain, old, ordinary ice rather than newer chemical recipes. The chemicals can super-cool and damage skin cells resulting in blistering or worse. Ice can only cool as low as 32° Fahrenheit, then it melts. As ice melts when contacting your skin, an insulating layer of water safely develops to disperse and buffer the cold. Ice is nice! One can conveniently place ice bags in a wide-mouth thermos and transport them to sporting events or workouts.

BRUISING

After the bleeding stops and our blood clots, the body knows what to do next. It must clean up that traffic accident—move the cars out of the way, sweep up the glass, etc. As our lymphatic system spreads out the cellular debris for transport away from the site of damage, we notice some surrounding bruising. The blood is spreading out, being brought to the surface so it can be absorbed and flushed away. The amount of bruising parallels the severity of initial bleeding and damage.

A doctor's duty requires him/her to estimate the extent of ligament damage and institute treatments which allow the frayed ends of moderate and severe ligament tears to over-lap for maximal healing. Sometimes I still apply a cast for third degree ankle sprains. I want the foot held in a neutral position for about 3 weeks so that the torn ends settle in apposition and scar can bond them in somewhat the same relationship as existed before the tear. For lesser, but painful, sprains (say first degree or second degree) you can stand some empty milk bottles under the covers at the foot of your bed to keep the heavy covers from twisting your foot as you sleeplessly search for a comfortable position. Obtain an x-ray if you suspect a significant injury. Sometimes a fracture (broken bone) may fool you. Swelling is not the only key for estimating the extent of involvement. A moderate sprain can bleed more than a small break. ("Break" and fracture are interchangeable words with the exact same meaning, contrary to some quizzical stares from confused patients.)

Recently, a long time patient and friend of mine gingerly walked into my office because his week old sprain wasn't improving. Bob certainly was not a "rookie" to injury as he played college football for Pittsburgh in his younger days. Despite rather minimal swelling, his x-rays confirmed a fracture of the 5th metatarsal (foot bone) notoriously known to heal slowly and with some difficulty. At times, surgery to place a screw across this fracture site is necessary. (Figure 16-L) His removable cast was planned for a 3 - 6 week interval dependent on the appearance of callous (healing bone) as

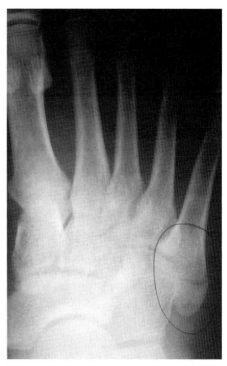

Figure 16-L: Fracture at base of fifth metatarsal

monitored by x-ray. He did heal by 7 weeks, and no surgery was required. If in doubt, obtain an x-ray.

HINTS

- **REST**—try to stay off the sprain. If third degree (severe), a splint or cast may be indicated.

- **ICE**—ice, ice, ice for 20 minutes every couple of hours. Use this for days until the angriness and warmth subside. **Be cautious about applying ice for long periods of time over the superficially located peroneal nerve that travels below the fibular head near the knee. I have seen or heard of three cases of foot drop lasting 2 to 3 months following prolonged ice.**

- **COMPRESSION**—it's o.k. to use an elastic wrap but don't get it uneven, wrinkled, or too tight. If your toes are swelling—the wrap is probably too tight. Definitely loosen it at night for sleeping—you might wake up with dead blue toes. Physical therapists have rehabilitation machines called Jobst compression units that sequentially compress your toes, ankle and leg to push the fluid out of the foot and down the leg.

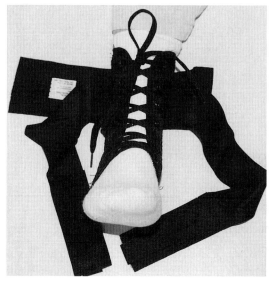

Figure 16-M: Lace-up ankle brace on foot — front view

• **ELEVATION**—move the hurt part higher than heart level. A footstool is not high enough. Use several pillows under the ankle at night.

• **ANTI-INFLAMMATORIES**—These are very effective at limiting the inflammatory problem we described as blood escapes into the surrounding tissues. Ibuprofen 400mg every 8 hours or Aleve 200mg every 12 hours are reasonable doses to use. Ingest it with meals and don't use these chemicals if there is a history of aspirin allergy, ulcers, liver problems, or if you are using blood-thinners. Tylenol is not an anti-inflammatory. Plain old aspirin is also effective (2 tablets every 6 - 8 hours) but is a bit more harsh on stomachs.

• **LACE-UP BRACES**—These are a great invention. Besides proving useful as an injury treatment, they

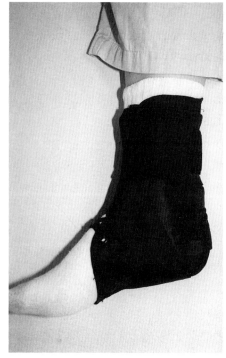

Figure 16-N: Lace-up ankle brace on foot — side view

may be then worn as a preventative support. Some colleges require all of their players to wear them in practice to diminish lost game days. They are more practical than taping. Even a well applied tape job will loosen by half-time. The lace-up braces achieve the effect of reapplication simply by tightening the laces. A highly skilled athletic trainer is not required for their application. The brace can be low profile enough to be worn with everyday laced shoes (probably not loafers). (Figure 16-M and Figure 16-N)

REHABILITATION

Once you are hurt, surrounding muscles receive negative messages and atrophy (shrink) out of reflex. We graphically see this demonstrated with knee injuries—the quadriceps (thigh) muscle just melts away. Our recovery efforts must also focus above and below the site of any injury. An ankle injury necessitates retraining the calf and anterior-lateral leg muscles. Therapists and trainers have established successful programs to regain tone. Another phenomenon now enters the recovery picture. Sorry for the big word but here it is—PROPRIOCEPTION. This means "position sense." When a basketball player jumps into the air to grab a rebound he doesn't have to look at his foot on the way down to be assured of properly landing onto the gym floor. He inherently knows whether he is off-balance or not. That feed-back from ankle and foot to brain is called position sense. These nerves are believed to travel along with the ankle ligaments. Guess what happens to these nerves if their neighbor, the ligament, is disrupted? My senior year in high school, I suffered a moderately severe ankle sprain and used the "milk bottle in bed" trick to allow sleep, so as to keep the weight of the covers from twisting and pressing against my sore swollen ankle. A rapid return to sport precipitated a second sprain and then a third sprain. Why so many in a short period of time? I hadn't allowed regrowth of my position sense nerves even though the ligament stability had reasonably recovered. Our physical therapy department easily demonstrates this gap in total recovery to "impatient patients." We simply ask an athlete with a badly sprained left ankle to balance on his right foot only, while closing his eyes. He/she can demonstrate reasonable athletic ability and not look like a "spaz." When they switch to the injured left ankle they flunk the test, immediately losing their balance. The brain hasn't received the proper response information to contract muscles rapidly. Trainers can help immensely by utilizing what superficially appear to be stupid, elementary, balancing and coordination drills. Once the athlete flunks our test, he senses our wisdom and becomes a believer. An ankle brace or tape increases the sensory input on our skin and enhances the transfer of this information to the brain. Therefore, tape works for two reasons—support and added sensory input. See a trainer for the specific balance exercises.

Chapter 17

The Martial Arts: How Safe?

Richard B. Birrer, M.D.

INTRODUCTION

The martial arts have recently emerged from a several thousand year history enshrouded in mystery and magic. This brutal activity generating a multitude of applications has burst upon the global scene. Commercial interests, health, self defense, fitness reasons, media hype, and international collaboration have attracted at least 75 million participants worldwide, with eight million devotees in America alone. Self-defense training, sports competition, self-confidence building, health and recreation, environmental and social support, conditioning and fitness, and philosophical, religious, and psychological transformation are the usual reasons for participating. In many locations worldwide the annual growth rate is expected to be 20% to 25%. Revenues probably exceed 250 million dollars yearly on an international basis.

As a combat art, the martial arts have traditionally represented a large number of offensive and defensive fighting techniques derived from the Far East. Historically, the techniques were originally developed in India and then transmitted to mainland China by Bodhidharma, the legendary founder of the famous Shaolin school. During the Sui and T'ang Dynasties these skills were spread to Korea and Okinawa and eventually to Japan, Indonesia, and the Philippines. Throughout most of these formative years the arts were secretly developed and transferred by word of mouth due, in large part, to repressive feudalism. Since World War II American servicemen carried the arts world-wide so that virtually everyone has been exposed to some aspect of the martial arts. Today, much of the exposure and hype bombards viewers through television, video, and cinema. The exploits of Bruce Lee, Jean-Claude Van Damme, and female heroes are clearly etched in the minds of many children and adults and have become synonymous with the combat warrior. Fortunately, the reality of the martial arts is far from this media presentation.

Traditionally, the term "martial arts" has referred to systems of attack and defense involving specialized weapons, protective equipment and battlefield use developed by and for professional groups of warriors for purposes of identity, unity, and survival. Outside battlefield situations, civilian forms evolved primarily as methods of self-defense, sports competition, or way of life. Generically, the term "martial arts" loosely refers to any of the fighting styles or systems of fighting techniques derived in whole or part from the Far East, utilizing one or more different body parts (i.e., hands, feet, elbow, knee, head, etc.) Jiu-jitsu, aikido, and judo are included, even though the International Judo Federation has designated judo as a sport and not a martial art. Weapon use may also be incorporated. As a matter of practicality, and due to the newness in the United States (only several hundred years of history), boxing has evolved as the "martial arts" form favored and practiced by Americans.

Thousands of different schools, systems, and styles exist, and many are associated with an infrastructure based on some form of eastern philosophy. Most teach unarmed self-defense techniques as well as the use of weaponry while incorporating a spiritual and philosophical component designed to psychologically transform the practitioner. The term "martial ways" primarily focuses on the psychological aspects with the combative components being secondary. "Martial disciplines" collectively refers to both the "martial ways" and the "fighting art." All successful systems incorporate some form of achievement designation. Typically, belt or sash color is used to identify skill level (lighter colors are used to denote less experienced while darker colors are reserved for more advanced levels of proficiency). Stripes and numbers (i.e., 10 = white [beginner] to 1 = black [advanced]) may also be used. Approximately 1 in 500 participants achieves the coveted level of black belt which is the basic departure point for advanced studies.

Despite the historically disciplined nature of the martial arts, their evolution, particularly in the United States, has been anything but disciplined. With the exception of Judo and Tae Kwon Do which are recognized Olympic sports, none of the other martial arts have standardized their rules and regulations to allow for consistency and comparability. There is no universal standard required for promotion, competition, training, or instructor quality. Going from one dojo or dojang to the next often results in having to re-establish proficiency levels and may lead to injury because of significant differences in training expectations, equipment, environmental conditions, or teaching staff competence. Dr. Birrer clearly remembers having to retest for his black belt after returning to the United States despite having achieved black belt status in the same style while overseas. In the United States commercial exploitation is often the underlying driving force preventing standardization and consolidation.

THE INJURY PROFILE

The martial arts can be hazardous activity. Over the last two decades a number of studies have attempted to investigate the type and extent of trauma in this sport. Dr. Birrer's research, the largest of these studies, involved some 15,000 international participants tracked over 18 years. The investigation was done by questionnaire and observation of training halls as well as tournaments. All martial arts including jiu-jitsu, aikido, and judo were studied and an effort was made to not only describe the type and extent of the injuries, but why they occur and what can be done to prevent them. The following represents a summary of what is currently known about the trauma epidemiology of the martial arts.

The average martial arts athlete practices 5.6 hours a week (range can be 40 hours/week for an Olympic athlete to less than 1 hour/week for non-competitive individuals in informal settings). About one-third of the time is spent outside the class in informal settings whereas the remaining two-thirds occurs in class. At least 47 countries in five continents have been studied in a wide variety of traditional and non-traditional styles: karatedo, tae kwon do, judo, gong-fu, taiji, kendo, arnis, eskrima, kempo, etc. The average age of female participants is about 19 years and for males about 21 years. 83% of participants are males and 17% are females with the difference widening in com-

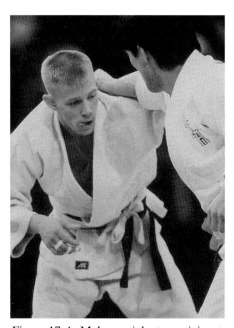

Figure 17-A: Male martial arts participant

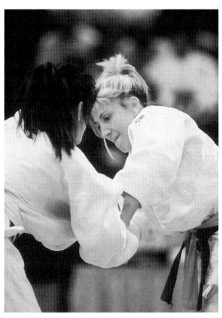

Figure 17-B: Lady martial arts participant

petitive situations. (Figure 17-A and Figure 17-B) Table #1 illustrates the common types of injuries and their degree of severity. (Figure 17-C) It is important to note that the least severe injuries are fortunately the most common. Table #2 shows where these injuries occur. (Figure 17-D) Note that most trauma occurs to the lower extremity (40%) especially leg, ankle, and foot/toes (29%). Thankfully, the fewest injuries occur to the neck (1%), but the head, face, and neck receive the harshest trauma. The type, pattern, and severity of injuries for males and females are the same before the age of ten;

TABLE # 1 NUMBER AND SEVERITY OF GENERIC INJURIES		
	PERCENT	SEVERITY
CONTUSIONS	43	1.30
SPRAINS/STRAINS	27	1.60
ABRASIONS/LACERATIONS	13	2.20
FRACTURES	6	3.70
DISLOCATIONS	5	3.80
MISCELLANEOUS	6	3.90
TOTAL	100	
AVERAGE		2.75

Figure 17-C: Table #1 — Number and severity of generic injuries

thereafter, both sexes suffer more frequent and serious injuries while certain injuries are gender specific (i.e., genital, breast, etc.). Fighting, particularly contact sparring, is the most common cause of injury in almost three-quarters of cases. (Figure 17-E) The rate and severity of injury is directly related to the amount of contact. Also, males are injured more frequently than females because males compete more often and appear to be more aggressive. In competitive situations, the head, lower extremity, and upper extremity are injured in that order. Interestingly enough,

TABLE # 2 NUMBER AND SEVERITY OF INJURIES BY ANATOMICAL SITE		
	PERCENT	SEVERITY
HEAD	3%	3.5
FACE	8%	3.8
NECK	1%	2.8
SHOULDER	5%	2.0
ELBOW	5%	1.7
ARM / FOREARM	6%	1.5
WRIST	6%	1.5
FINGERS / HAND	11%	1.9
TRUNK	7%	1.4
GROIN	8%	2.6
HIP	3%	1.2
KNEE	4%	1.8
THIGH / LEG	17%	1.5
ANKLE	2%	1.6
FOOT / TOES	14%	1.7
TOTAL	100%	
AVERAGE		2.03

Figure 17-D: Table #2 — Number and severity of injuries by anatomical site

TABLE # 3 NUMBER AND SEVERITY OF INJURIES BY ACTIVITY		
	PERCENT	SEVERITY
FIGHTING	74	2.10
FORMS	5	1.30
WEAPONS	2	1.60
BASICS	14	1.50
MISCELLANEOUS	5	2.30
TOTAL	100	
AVERAGE		1.76

Figure 17-E: Table #3 — Number and severity of injuries by activity

while the expected defender is hurt 70% of the time the attacker is injured at least 20% and may be more seriously injured than the defender. In 8% of situations both are simultaneously injured. As might be expected, the vast majority of these injuries occur in the setting of no protective equipment. Also, lack of supervision (i.e., informal training settings) is associated with a greater likelihood and severity of trauma. Breakage and weapon usage are associated with injury, although infrequently. Whereas the degree of injury is mild during weapon usage, the severity of trauma during breakage is often severe (e.g., concussion, fracture, puncture, and laceration wounds).

Approximately 70% of injured participants recuperate quickly without training interruption. However, 30% suffer significant measurable amounts of disability. Yet, almost 85% of all participants do not seek medical assistance following injury and only slightly more than 30% report their injury to their instructor or health care professional! Very often injury occurrence is not observed despite the presence of supervision. Instructors would be encouraged to study this book as knowledge of injury mechanism serves as a foundation for injury recognition.

What is the risk of serious injury? Severe trauma does occur in the martial arts. Cerebral concussion occurs five times more commonly than long bone fracture. Life threatening injury demanding prompt and aggressive medical management fortunately is rare—125 injuries per 100,000 participants/year. Regrettably, fatalities have been reported following a blow or kick to the chest, head, or neck.

The highest rate and severity of injury parallels the level of experience. The lower (color) belt ranks (inexperience) and younger age groups (immaturity) are associated with increased risk of trauma. Less than one year of training and introduction into tournament/competitive situations strongly correlates to increased injury risk. The chance of reinjury appears to be directly related to participation in tournaments, contact sparring, unfamiliar settings, and lack of protective gear. A lack of medical support, rehabilitation, supervision, qualified medical staff, and premature return to training create the scenario for trouble. Most tournament settings have no formal arrangements for physician coverage. In contrast, boxing matches must have a ringside physician present by wise legislation enforced by USA Boxing. Wrestling tournaments at least utilize high school athletic trainers for advice and consultation.

Certain martial art styles are associated with particular injury patterns. Tae kwon do is characterized by increased amounts of lower extremity and head trauma. Kendo is associated with a predominance of left side injuries. Karate styles emphasizing predominantly upper body techniques have proportionately increased numbers of upper extremity injuries. Judo has proportionately increased numbers of upper extremity injuries. Judo, jiu-jitsu, and aikido have an increased percentage of shoulder and ligamentous injuries.

SUMMARY

1. There is **significant risk** of injury in the martial arts that is cumulative.

2. The majority of injuries are **categorized** as mild to moderate in severity.

3. The majority of **injury types** are contusions, sprains, strains, cuts, and abrasions.

4. The most commonly injured **area** is the lower extremity, particularly the leg; the least is the neck.

5. The **mildest** injuries occur to the arm/forearm; the **most severe** to the face and head.

6. The **majority** of all injuries occurs during fighting, particularly during **non-competitive training** situations.

7. **Protective equipment** significantly reduces injury rate and severity.

8. **Experience** is associated with fewer injuries that are less severe.

9. **Males** experience more injuries and of higher severity than females.

10. The majority of injuries are **overlooked** and not reported.

11. **Increasing** levels of **contact** during fighting are directly associated with increasing rates and severity of injury.

12. The risk of **life threatening** injury is very small: 1 in 500 to 600 injuries.

13. The percentage chance of injury during **competition** is greater than that of non-competition, and the **severity** of trauma is higher during tournaments.

RISK FACTORS

1. Failure to use protective equipment regularly

2. Lack of experience

3. Male gender

4. Competition

5. Lack of supervision

RECOMMENDATIONS

1. Regularly use protective equipment.

2. Train under safe conditions—clean, well-lit environment.

3. Expect that injury may occur but seek medical assistance for any injury that interferes with training because of pain or disability.

4. Train with an instructor who is certified to teach the martial arts, and who is safety certified (American Red Cross, etc.).

5. Avoid informal sparring situations.

6. Seek to establish medical supervision of high risk tournaments. Seek the services of a ringside physician. Study the safety recommendations of USA Boxing. Suggest that your physician review this text as a concise, current reference.

CONCLUSION

Under optimal conditions males and females, young and old, can safely participate in the martial arts for health, sport, and safety reasons. While injuries do occur, serious trauma is the exception and not the rule. As a matter of fact, when the safety of the martial arts is compared to other recreational and sports activities, it is ranked sixteenth in a field of twenty. Specifically, the martial arts have an injury rate one-twentieth that of football and appears to be safer than golf and general exercise. Certainly, a high level of fitness and skill may be achieved by regular participation in the martial arts with an awareness of safety considerations.

Chapter 18

Pre and Post Competition Exams

PRE-COMPETITION HISTORY AND PHYSICAL

As a guest, I recently attended an out-of-state "Reality" fighting tournament sponsored by a friend and respected former instructor. Arriving a day early, I offered to assist as needed. With my out-of-state status, a locally licensed physician was hired to "officially" function as tournament physician. I was appalled to learn that no pre-bout history and physical exams were planned. The local doctor had never before covered a karate or boxing competition and planned to show up 30 minutes prior to the 12 bouts. Sensing an opportunity to provide assistance, I volunteered to perform the pre-bout exams during their mid-afternoon weigh-ins. With needless delay to the nervous, hungry athletes, some old forms from a prior tournament were photocopied at the last minute. The competitors and coaches griped that this disorganized, spur-of-the-moment "paper work" and physicals created a hardship. In a perfect scenario a professionally designed, specialized history form (Competitor Medical Questionnaire) could have been more efficiently mailed to each participant upon receipt of his application. (Figure 18-A) These exams demand a sophistication that is "sport specific" since a fighter is exposed to training and competitive injuries far different than those of a cross-country runner, basketball player, or cheerleader.

That night, we actually had to delay several bouts since some competitors decided to skip the afternoon exams. Ready to go and warmed-up, a less than ideal last minute locker room evaluation was performed. Were the physicals a waste of time? Absolutely not! I'll provide two specific examples. One competitor was not allowed to participate as he presented with patches of one day old, active, oozing, herpes simplex blisters around his mouth. He graciously accepted withdrawing when I explained to him that during his "anything-goes" fight, he risked the chance of blindness to himself and opponent should the virus infect the cornea. (See chapter on herpes).

A second competitor presented with a permanently dilated pupil present since his college football days. He was cleared by me to safely compete. The point of this story relates to critical decision-making if injury did occur and this defect not recognized pre-bout and noted on his medical record. If this competitor had been knocked-out (as happened to a martial artist in bout #2 that night), his dilated pupil would have been mistakenly attributed to serious concussive brain injury—a medical emergency. He would have possibly endured the cost of ambulance transportation to a hospital, admission, and a $1,000.00 brain scan. Pre-bout awareness of this existing abnormality would greatly simplify his life.

Pre-bout exams are absolute necessities. (Figure 18-B Physician's Pre-Bout Examination form.) You wouldn't believe the injuries and conditions that I have uncovered during this productive time with the athletes. Broken ribs, broken hands, recent concussions, hypertension, ruptured eardrums, fevers, swollen knees, positive HIV, and infectious skin diseases have all been casualties and discoveries of my pre-bout exam experiences. A great friend and mentor, Dr. Necip Ari, once alertly discovered an abdominal mass in a teenage boxer who confided about stomach pain. His life was saved as resultant exams revealed an abdominal cancer.

I will never forget being handed a crumpled-up piece of prescription pad paper after I had o.k.'d a 28 year old, first time competitor. The note originated from the family doctor of this **seizure** patient who recently and insanely decided to take-up the sport of boxing. His doctor naively reasoned that his seizures were well controlled on two medications. Talk about **my** being saved by a last minute bell. Never did this condition surface until he casually mentioned the note. (See how important a medical history becomes!) Never would he compete with my medical license at risk—an absolute contraindication to competitive boxing. His need to exercise was satisfied by informing him about aerobic boxing—same skills and benefits but no contact. He can go find other competitive pursuits.

The privately performed physical exam also gives athletes with last minute "cold feet" an honorable way to escape. I am "honored" to provide a "face-saving" mechanism for an uneasy competitor. Inwardly they signal for me to make it "The doctor wouldn't let me fight" and that's o.k. by me. I've still performed a service that will remain a well kept secret.

A tournament director and a ringside physician can prevent potential miscommunication by utilization of the Physician's Post-Bout Examination Form for injuries identified during or after a competition (Figure 18-C). Make it a rule that each competitor must see the doctor as he leaves the ring. These forms concisely detail information regarding a recognized injury situation and confirm appropriate instructions for medical follow-up and activity modification. All parties now are informed and notified in writing.

Organize yourself and your tournament. Obtain histories early so that each competitor carries the history form to the doctor's physical exam. This exam can now proceed with special emphasis on identified problems. If your doctor has knowledge of problem areas, his exam is greatly elevated in usefulness. If no information is shared, the exam becomes a "veterinary" exercise. (Figure 18-D) Horses, dogs, and cats can't tell you what's wrong with them. Fully utilize gifts of communication to elevate the level of sophistication.

BOXERGENICS™ PRESS©
SPORTS SCIENCE CENTRE
335 BILLINGSLEY ROAD
CHARLOTTE, NC   28211

TELEPHONE: (704) 334-4663   FAX: (704) 343-0811   TOLL FREE: 1-800-774-6284

COMPETITOR MEDICAL QUESTIONNAIRE

Name:_____ Date of Birth:_____ Today's Date:_____
Address:_____ Telephone:_____
Emergency Contact:_____ Telephone:_____
No. Bouts/Competitions_____ Wins____/Losses____ No. Times Been KO'd_____

MEDICAL HISTORY:	NO	YES
•Medicine Allergy? List:_____	❏	❏
•List Medicines/Drugs Used:_____	❏	❏
•Any Substance Abuse (Drugs, Tobacco, Alcohol)	❏	❏
•Prior Surgery? List Type & Dates_____	❏	❏
•Overnight Hospitalizations? List Reason & Dates_____	❏	❏
•Recommended Evaluations such as Scans, X-rays, EKG, EEG, Stress Tests? If yes, List	❏	❏
_____		
•Do you currently have any "Training Injuries" to discuss?	❏	❏
•Have you had any missed Training Sessions in the past three weeks?	❏	❏

▲▽

HEENT:	NO	YES	EXTREMITIES:	NO	YES
•Ever been knocked out/"bell rung"/been unconscious/suffered a concussion? (Including childhood injuries)	❏	❏	•Ever broken (fractured) a bone or had a cast? List Location & Date _____	❏	❏
•Ever had a seizure/fit/convulsion?	❏	❏	•Severe sprain/torn ligament/injured joint?	❏	❏
•Recent headaches/dizziness/impaired memory?	❏	❏	•Swollen joints?	❏	❏
•Double vision/blurred vision?	❏	❏	•Spinal injury or ruptured discs?	❏	❏
•Retinal detachment?	❏	❏			
•Glasses or contact lenses?	❏	❏	**SYSTEMIC:**		
•Vision much worse in one eye than other?	❏	❏			
•Hearing difficulty or ruptured eardrum?	❏	❏	•Diabetes?	❏	❏
•Broken nose?	❏	❏	•Bleeding disorder/poor clotting?	❏	❏
•Recent sore throat?	❏	❏	•Hepatitis?	❏	❏
•Cold sores/fever blisters/herpes simplex?	❏	❏	•HIV/AIDS		
			•Close relative dying before age 50 of heart disease/unknown causes?	❏	❏
HEART/LUNGS:			•Recent fever/chills?	❏	❏
•Fainted while exercising?	❏	❏	**ABDOMEN:**		
•Chest pain/heart murmur/irregular heart beat?	❏	❏	•Hernia/rupture?	❏	❏
•High blood pressure/rheumatic or scarlet fever?	❏	❏	•Single kidney/single testicle?	❏	❏
•Asthma/bronchitis/T.B./wheezing?	❏	❏	•Blood in urine?	❏	❏
•Heat stroke/heat exhaustion?	❏	❏	•Vomiting/Diarrhea in past 3 weeks?	❏	❏

FEMALES:	NO	YES	
			▲▽▲▽▲▽▲▽▲▽▲▽▲▽▲▽▲▽▲▽▲▽▲▽▲▽
•Are you pregnant?	❏	❏	Physician's Name:_____
•Regular menstruation?	❏	❏	Address:_____
•Have you missed a period?	❏	❏	_____
			Telephone:_____

▲▽

I HEREBY STATE THAT, TO THE BEST OF MY
KNOWLEDGE, MY ANSWERS TO THE ABOVE
QUESTIONS ARE CORRECT.

_____Date: _____
Athlete's Signature

_____Date:_____
Parent/Guardian Signature (if athlete is a minor)

Figure 18-A: Competitor Medical Questionnaire form

BOXERGENICS™ PRESS©
SPORTS SCIENCE CENTRE
335 BILLINGSLEY ROAD
CHARLOTTE, NC 28211

TELEPHONE: (704) 334-4663   FAX: (704) 343-0811   TOLL FREE: 1-800-774-6284

PHYSICIAN'S PRE-BOUT EXAMINATION

Name:_____ Date of Birth:_____ Today's Date:_____

B.P. _____   Height _____   Vision (Optional) Right: 20/_____

Pulse _____   Weight _____   Left: 20/_____

❖❖❖

	NORMAL	ABNORMAL
HEENT:		
Alert	❏	❏
PERRL	❏	❏
Visual Fields	❏	❏
Nasal/Facial tenderness	❏	❏
Hearing	❏	❏
Neck supple	❏	❏
Dental Hygiene and TMJ	❏	❏
Nodes	❏	❏
Good Balance with Eyes closed (15 Seconds)	❏	❏
Finger-to-Nose test	❏	❏
HEART & LUNG:		
Lungs clear	❏	❏
Ribs non-tender to A-P/Lateral Compression	❏	❏
No murmurs or irregular beats	❏	❏
ABDOMEN:		
Non-tender	❏	❏
No masses	❏	❏
No hernias or Testicular Abnormality (by history)	❏	❏
No organomegaly	❏	❏
EXTREMITIES:		
Full squat and duck walk (heels/ankles)	❏	❏
Touches toes (spine)	❏	❏
Full shoulder rotation	❏	❏
Elbows fully extend	❏	❏
Wrists and hands (extended/clenched)	❏	❏
Toes and feet	❏	❏
SKIN:		
Herpes Simplex	❏	❏
Impetigo	❏	❏
Rashes	❏	❏
Lacerations	❏	❏

❖❖❖

CLEARED_____   NOT CLEARED * _____   Physician's Name:_____

* REASON_____ Address:_____

                                                        _____

PHYSICIAN SIGNATURE:_____   Telephone:_____

Figure 18-B: Physician's Pre-Bout Examination form

BOXERGENICS™ PRESS©
SPORTS SCIENCE CENTRE
335 BILLINGSLEY ROAD
CHARLOTTE, NORTH CAROLINA 28001
TELEPHONE: (704) 334-4663   FAX: (704) 343-0811   TOLL FREE: 1-800-774-6284

PHYSICIAN'S POST-BOUT
MEDICAL REPORT

DATE:_____

Event:_____ Location:_____

Name:_____ Age:_____ Wt. Class:_____

Address:_____

_____Telephone:_____

❖❖❖

Mechanism of Injury:_____

_____

Physical Findings:_____

_____

_____

Impression:_____

_____

Initial Treatment:_____

_____

_____

❖❖❖

RECOMMENDATIONS

❑ Fitness Training Only (No Contact)   ❑ No Practice

❑ No Competition   ❑ Emergency Room Evaluation

❑ Non-Emergency Physician Follow-Up: _____Days / _____Weeks

❑ Restriction: ○ 30 Days   ○ 90 Days   ○ 180 Days   ○ _____ Days

Physician's Signature:_____ Date:_____

Physician's Address:_____

Telephone Number:_____

Athlete's Signature:_____ Date:_____

Figure 18-C: Physician's Post-Bout Examination form

NOTICE TO PARTICIPANTS©:

IT IS THE RESPONSIBILITY OF THE ATHLETE TO INFORM HIS/HER COACH AND THE RINGSIDE PHYSICIAN (PRE-BOUT PHYSICAL) OF ANY PHYSICAL CONDITION(S) OR PROBLEMS WHICH COULD AFFECT THE WELL-BEING OR PERFORMANCE OF THE COMPETITOR AND HIS/HER OPPONENTS.

AVAILABLE THROUGH:
BOXERGENICS™ PRESS, 335 BILLINGSLEY ROAD, CHARLOTTE, NC 28211
TELEPHONE: (704) 334-4663   FAX: (704) 343-0811   TOLL FREE: 1-800-774-6284

Figure 18-D: Notice to Participants

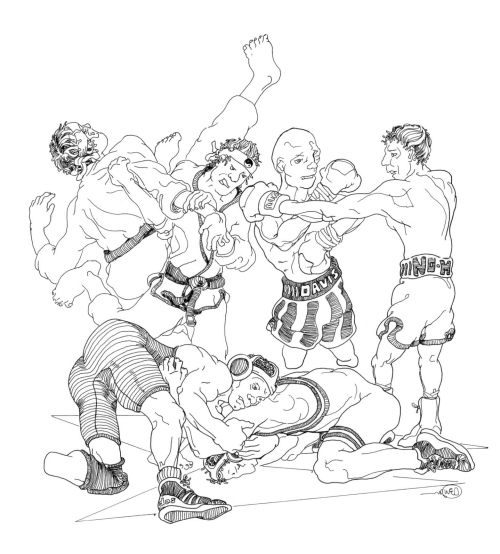

Index

NOTES

NOTES

NOTES

NOTES

NOTES

INJURY LOG

INJURY LOG

REHAB GOALS

REHAB GOALS

NOW AVAILABLE FROM BOXERGENICS™ PRESS

BX-1: *BOXERGENICS™ VIDEO*—The first medically designed boxing aerobic workout to promote overall fitness, symmetry, confidence, and well-being . .**$19.95**

BX-2: *SPORTSMEDICINE FOR THE COMBAT ARTS*—Provides a thorough understanding of injuries sustained by all those participating in martial arts, boxing, grappling, wrestling, and law enforcement training **$24.95**

BX-3: *BOXERGENICS™ T-SHIRT*—*"No Matter What ..."*—Sizes available— M, L, XL—Colors available—White, Red, Yellow **$15.00**

GG-1: *THE GRAPPLING GLOVE™*—The original glove custom designed to the needs of the grappler. Worn on world-wide pay-per-view by the "Reality" fighters of Ultimate Fighting Championship and Battlecade Extreme Fighting, pictured on page 68—Sizes available—M, L, XL . . . . **Pair—$49.95**

HW-1: *COREPAD™ HANDWRAP*—A modern, customized slip-on handwrap, physician designed, utilizing modern biomaterials to protect the hand and wrist, pictured on page 58. Sizes available—S, M, L, XL . . . .**Call for Price**

PE-1: *COMPETITOR MEDICAL QUESTIONNAIRE*—Two part carbonless form. See Chapter 18 (Page 262) . . . .**Packs of 25—$9.95**

PE-2: *PHYSICIAN'S PRE-BOUT EXAMINATION FORM*—Two part carbonless form. See Chapter 18 (Page 263) . . . .**Packs of 25—$9.95**

PE-3: *PHYSICIAN'S POST-BOUT EXAMINATION FORM*—Three part carbonless form. See Chapter 18 (Page 264) . . . .**Packs of 25—$10.95**

PE-4: *NOTICE TO ALL PARTICIPANTS CHART*—Recommended for physicians/promoters. Fits easily in briefcase. Laminated, 12"X16". See Chapter 18 (Page 265) . . . .**Each—$8.95**

PE-5: *HEAD INJURY SAFETY GUIDELINES CHART*—A must for all gyms, training studios, etc. Promotes head injury safety awareness. Laminated, 24" X 36". See Chapter 8 (Page 139) . . . .**Each—$12.95**

IC-1: *WOMEN'S AWARENESS RESPONSE* (**The self-defense book for women**)—By Irwin Carmichael—Developed by actual interviews with convicted rapists, robbers, and molesters of women. 73 photographs and 112 pages **$14.95**

BX-1   **BX-2**   **BX-3/Size_____/Color_____**

PE-1   **PE-2**   **PE-3**   **PE-4**   **PE-5**   **IC-1**

GG-1/Size_____   **HW-1/Size_____**

Name_____

Address _____

City_____ST____Zip ____

Credit Card # _____

Visa____MasterCard____Exp. Date _____

Signature _____

Shipping & Handling $4.95 for first item and $1.00 for each additional item*. NC residents include 6% sales tax.

SUB-TOTAL_____
S & H_____
NC TAX_____
TOTAL_____

Mail form to:
Boxergenics™ Press
335 Billingsley Road
Charlotte, NC 28211

Or call 1-800-774-6284 to place order
* Allow 3 to 6 weeks for shipping.
http://www.concordnc.com/boxergenics

NOW AVAILABLE FROM BOXERGENICS™ PRESS

BX-1: *BOXERGENICS™ VIDEO*—The first medically designed boxing aerobic workout to promote overall fitness, symmetry, confidence, and well-being . .**$19.95**

BX-2: *SPORTSMEDICINE FOR THE COMBAT ARTS*—Provides a thorough understanding of injuries sustained by all those participating in martial arts, boxing, grappling, wrestling, and law enforcement training **$24.95**

BX-3: *BOXERGENICS™ T-SHIRT—"No Matter What ..."*—Sizes available— M, L, XL—Colors available—White, Red, Yellow **$15.00**

GG-1: *THE GRAPPLING GLOVE™*—The original glove custom designed to the needs of the grappler. Worn on world-wide pay-per-view by the "Reality" fighters of Ultimate Fighting Championship and Battlecade Extreme Fighting, pictured on page 68—Sizes available—M, L, XL . . . . **Pair—$49.95**

HW-1: *COREPAD™ HANDWRAP*—A modern, customized slip-on handwrap, physician designed, utilizing modern biomaterials to protect the hand and wrist, pictured on page 58. Sizes available—S, M, L, XL . . . .**Call for Price**

PE-1: *COMPETITOR MEDICAL QUESTIONNAIRE*—Two part carbonless form. See Chapter 18 (Page 262) . . . .**Packs of 25—$9.95**

PE-2: *PHYSICIAN'S PRE-BOUT EXAMINATION FORM*—Two part carbonless form. See Chapter 18 (Page 263) . . . .**Packs of 25—$9.95**

PE-3: *PHYSICIAN'S POST-BOUT EXAMINATION FORM*—Three part carbonless form. See Chapter 18 (Page 264) . . . .**Packs of 25—$10.95**

PE-4: *NOTICE TO ALL PARTICIPANTS CHART*—Recommended for physicians/promoters. Fits easily in briefcase. Laminated, 12"X16". See Chapter 18 (Page 265) . . . .**Each—$8.95**

PE-5: *HEAD INJURY SAFETY GUIDELINES CHART*—A must for all gyms, training studios, etc. Promotes head injury safety awareness. Laminated, 24" X 36". See Chapter 8 (Page 139) . . . .**Each—$12.95**

IC-1: *WOMEN'S AWARENESS RESPONSE* **(The self-defense book for women)**—By Irwin Carmichael—Developed by actual interviews with convicted rapists, robbers, and molesters of women. 73 photographs and 112 pages **$14.95**

BX-1   BX-2   BX-3/Size_____ /Color_____   Shipping & Handling $4.95 for first item and $1.00 for each additional item*.

PE-1   PE-2   PE-3   PE-4   PE-5   IC-1   NC residents include 6% sales tax.

GG-1/Size_____   HW-1/Size_____

Name_____

Address _____

City_____ST____Zip ____

Credit Card # _____

Visa____MasterCard____Exp. Date _____

Signature _____

SUB-TOTAL_____

S & H_____

NC TAX_____

TOTAL_____

Mail form to:

Boxergenics™ Press
335 Billingsley Road
Charlotte, NC 28211

Or call 1-800-774-6284 to place order
* Allow 3 to 6 weeks for shipping.
http://www.concordnc.com/boxergenics

NOW AVAILABLE FROM BOXERGENICS™ PRESS

BX-1: *BOXERGENICS™ VIDEO*—The first medically designed boxing aerobic workout to promote overall fitness, symmetry, confidence, and well-being . .**$19.95**

BX-2: *SPORTSMEDICINE FOR THE COMBAT ARTS*—Provides a thorough understanding of injuries sustained by all those participating in martial arts, boxing, grappling, wrestling, and law enforcement training **$24.95**

BX-3: *BOXERGENICS™ T-SHIRT—"No Matter What ..."*—Sizes available—M, L, XL—Colors available—White, Red, Yellow **$15.00**

GG-1: *THE GRAPPLING GLOVE™*—The original glove custom designed to the needs of the grappler. Worn on world-wide pay-per-view by the "Reality" fighters of Ultimate Fighting Championship and Battlecade Extreme Fighting, pictured on page 68—Sizes available—M, L, XL . . . . **Pair—$49.95**

HW-1: *COREPAD™ HANDWRAP*—A modern, customized slip-on handwrap, physician designed, utilizing modern biomaterials to protect the hand and wrist, pictured on page 58. Sizes available—S, M, L, XL . . . .**Call for Price**

PE-1: *COMPETITOR MEDICAL QUESTIONNAIRE*—Two part carbonless form. See Chapter 18 (Page 262) . . . .**Packs of 25—$9.95**

PE-2: *PHYSICIAN'S PRE-BOUT EXAMINATION FORM*—Two part carbonless form. See Chapter 18 (Page 263) . . . .**Packs of 25—$9.95**

PE-3: *PHYSICIAN'S POST-BOUT EXAMINATION FORM*—Three part carbonless form. See Chapter 18 (Page 264) . . . .**Packs of 25—$10.95**

PE-4: *NOTICE TO ALL PARTICIPANTS CHART*—Recommended for physicians/promoters. Fits easily in briefcase. Laminated, 12"X16". See Chapter 18 (Page 265) . . . .**Each—$8.95**

PE-5: *HEAD INJURY SAFETY GUIDELINES CHART*—A must for all gyms, training studios, etc. Promotes head injury safety awareness. Laminated, 24" X 36". See Chapter 8 (Page 139) . . . .**Each—$12.95**

IC-1: *WOMEN'S AWARENESS RESPONSE* **(The self-defense book for women)**—By Irwin Carmichael—Developed by actual interviews with convicted rapists, robbers, and molesters of women. 73 photographs and 112 pages **$14.95**

BX-1   BX-2   BX-3/Size_____ /Color_____

PE-1   PE-2   PE-3   PE-4   PE-5   IC-1

GG-1/Size_____   HW-1/Size_____

Name_____

Address _____

City_____ST____Zip ____

Credit Card # _____

Visa____MasterCard____Exp. Date _____

Signature _____

740519

Shipping & Handling $4.95 for first item and $1.00 for each additional item*.
NC residents include 6% sales tax.

SUB-TOTAL_____
S & H_____
NC TAX_____
TOTAL_____

Mail form to:
Boxergenics™ Press
335 Billingsley Road
Charlotte, NC 28211

Or call 1-800-774-6284 to place order
* Allow 3 to 6 weeks for shipping.
http://www.concordnc.com/boxergenics

BUSINESS/SCIENCE/TECHNOLOGY DIVISION
CHICAGO PUBLIC LIBRARY
400 SOUTH STATE STREET
CHICAGO, IL 60605

CHICAGO PUBLIC LIBRARY

R01212 11104

SportsMedicine
for the
Combat Arts

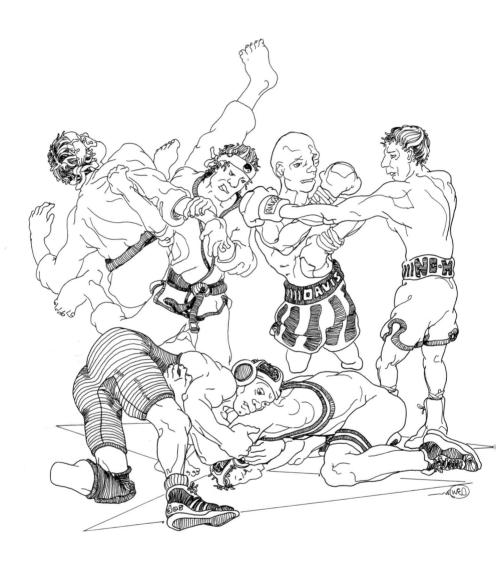